Sexual Magick

by Katon Shu'al

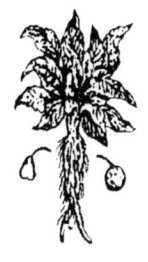

Mandrake of Oxford

Dedicated to Shantidevi-Nath 93

Mandrake of Oxford
Po Box 250
Oxford Ox1 1ap

ISBN 1 869928 40 7
3rd Edition 1995

All Rights Reserved © Katon Shu'al
& Mandrake *of Oxford*

*Cover design by Mogg Morgan,
based on a photograph by Michael R Goss*

also by Katon Shu'al
A Magician's Guide to Hindu Tantrik Sources
Medicine of the Gods - Basic principles of Ayurvedic medicine
The Tantrik knuckle-bone oracle (forthcoming)

Printed in Great Britain by
Antony Rowe Ltd, Chippenham, Wiltshire

Contents

Preface by Peter Redgrove v
Introduction vi
1. **Sexual Magick** 9
   Karezza and sexual vampirism 14
   A ritual interlude - Lopamudra 16
   Sex and the Hermetic Order of the Golden Dawn 23
   Three spirits in a chamber 33
   The licence to depart 38
   Homosexuality 40
   The magical importance of homosexuality 43
   Sexual magick today 44

2. **Serpent power** 50
   How many chakras are there? 52
   Some correspondences of the six chakras 57
   Common experience of the chakras 60
   Yogic techniques 61
   Symbolic arousal 62
   The Kamarupa temple meditation 64
   The Kalas 70
   Kundalini and Wilhelm Reich 72

3. **As Brothers Fight Ye!** 76
   Mysteries of Seth 76
   The Third Sex 95

4. **The Erotic Landscape** 98
   Appendix - woman to woman 110
   Bibliography & Index 112

Preface to second edition

I found it an inspiring experience recently when I gave a talk to a society composed largely of Thelemites. There was an atmosphere which is rare in purely literary or academic worlds. Readers of my *Black Goddess and the Sixth Sense* will know I regard the perception of atmosphere as very important. This one was complex, but I identified is as a fizz in the air exhaled by people who did not believe in the Fall. Or, to put it another way, the meeting had the fragrance of people who were on their way to solving their religious and sexual problems and happy that these turned out to be the same thing.

Sexual Magick has the same inspiring atmosphere, with the heart of the gnosis given on pages fourty-four to fourty-nine. Sex is a sacrament and crossing over into other modes of consciousness. It is the central act of the great work of transforming consciousness and through consciousness the world. Katon Shu'al recalls to us not only this essential foundation of magick, and its starting point for most adults, but that the original and natural conditions of life is magical. Sex, which was supposed to have caused the Fall, in fact can restore an Eden. It is neglect and ignorance of sex which is the Fall.

A valuable feature of Katon Shu'al's book is that he is non-sexist and reminds us that it is love which transforms, whatever the gender of the partners. I wish the book were longer, and that he had written much more on heterosexual, homosexual and auto-erotic magick in the same terms for he says: '. . . the first and perhaps most significant step is to start viewing one's sexuality as magical and allow all things to reinforce this intention. Thus any sexual act is also a magical ritual.' And so the rooms of such societies as have taken this step fill with the good atmosphere of people who are simultaneously sexual and spiritual and whose works are living under will.

Peter Redgrove.

Introduction

Love! and do what thou Wilt[1]

Sexual Magick is a very glamorous title for a book. Sexuality is often held up as the key to magick, which indeed it can be. However, nothing in magick is as simple as the mere turning of a key in a lock. Like sex itself, it needs maturity, sensitivity and dare I say it, training. Before you can really hope to make any of the ideas or techniques in this book work for you, you need to undertake the standard training of the magician. By all means read it, the words are for all, I hope it will inspire you to learn more about our ancient and venerable craft of magick. It is possible to learn magick from a book and indeed there are many good primers available now on the market.[2] But it is my sincere hope that over the next few years the traditional magical 'institution' of teaching passed freely from teacher to student will again establish itself in every land, as it was in the past.

This book started as a collection of talks and articles on related themes, written over the last few years. An earlier version of the first three chapters appeared in the pages of *Nuit-Isis* magazine, but the final three have never been published before but were written as workshop material for the Second National Symposium of Thelemic Magick, the Oxfordshire Pagan Fellowship and the Leeds University Union Occult Society (the latter two organisations now sadly disbanded).

These essays are about magick, an expression that has often been misunderstood, sometimes deliberately. Despite its many detractors, magick is an important, arguably even essential, element in every culture. The magician's life should, in an ideal world, be focused on one thing, the obtaining of knowledge. In the process he or she may

---

[1] 'Ama, et fac quod vis' attributed to Augustus of Hippo. At the risk of being called revisionist, this phrase seems to sum up all that is necessary in the Thelemic system without talk of any law.
[2] Free advice on starting in magick is available from the Oxford Golden Dawn Occult Society, C/O PO Box 250, Oxford, OX1 1AP (UK)

accumulate certain abilities or powers to change both themselves and their environments, but this is a sideline and the least important aspect of being a magician. Unlike most modern philosophers, magicians are interested in the fundamental meaning of life. Magick proposes a practical or yogic manner in which to gain this mystical knowledge and central to this method is the use of ritual. What we seek comes gradually.

Some of the magical techniques described below are admittedly only a part of a wide spectrum of magical activities. A few years ago it was fashionable, even amongst people who claimed to be pagans and therefore ought to have known better, to call the kind of magick discussed here 'black' magick. However, things move on and the pagan community has realised the danger of joining in a witch-hunt against some of its own minorities. In fact, fewer and fewer magical people are willing to accept the label 'white' magician or witch, as this in turn accepts the loaded argument that there exist the black variety who are in some way 'evil'. The people who set this agenda in the first place have been exposed as fundamentalist Christians who have a vested interesting in besmirching the reputation of *all* pagans, witches and magicians but realised that in order to do this they needed first to divide the community.

Incidentally, the term 'black' magick is probably a reference to the black arts of ancient Egypt which was sometimes called the land of black soil. It therefore has no real moral connotation any more than does the more accurate term 'left hand path'. Some pagans have even detected an element of racism in all this talk of black and white.

Western magick as it is practised now is eclectic in its approach. That is to say it borrows ideas and techniques from a wide range of global traditions. This symbiosis has been going on for so long it is almost impossible to point to a so-called native British tradition, should one want to. Even if one were to go back to the Celtic/shamanistic roots one finds links with the cultures of India and the Mediterranean. Contrary to the beliefs of some present day occultists, it is this long standing symbiosis which is the strength of modern magick.

During this century the influence of tantrik ideas from the Indian sub-continent has been particularly strong. The word 'Tantra' has a number of related meanings such as 'tradition' or 'treatise' and as such is similar in meaning to more familiar terms such as Kabbalah, grimoire or even magick. Words such as 'karma', 'dharma', and 'tattva', which stem from the Tantrik and Hindu tradition, have entered the magical vocabulary even of those who deny that the Eastern 'dharma' or 'yoga' is for us! The belief that Eastern ideas are not suitable for the westerner is clearly nonsense and can only be sustained by extreme parochialism and an ignorance of magical history. As Aleister Crowley was quick to point out, Eastern ideas have always found a fertile home in the West, and the prime example of this is the success of the essentially Eastern cult of Judeo-Christianity.

The now legendary *Hermetic Order of the Golden Dawn* and its precursor the *Theosophical Society* introduced countless new techniques gleaned from the Tantrik tradition, although often without proper acknowledgement. A charitable explanation of this might be that the leaders of these groups thought that if they named their sources prejudice would stop people experimenting.

Aleister Crowley was and continues to be one of the greatest influences on modern magick. Again this often goes unacknowledged, especially by supposed experts of the self styled 'new age' type. One of his achievements was in alerting us to the importance of certain Tantrik techniques, especially those that revolved around the mysteries of sex and sexuality and that sometimes go under the title of the left hand path.[3] Our debt to Aleister Crowley is immense, and his life and work figures large in the pages of what follows.

Katon Shual
Oxford 1994 ce

---

[3] The term has nothing to do with 'evil' practices but seems to originate from the magic associated with the left or more 'occult' face of the god Shiva.

Chapter 1
Sexual magick

Sexual magick is often considered to be a specialism within the greater magical tradition. Perhaps this is how it should be, in fact, earlier editions of this book were sometimes classified as 'advanced magical arts'. Perhaps I should say that for me, magick is a spiritual endeavour. Magick has been defined many times, most usefully by Aleister Crowley. To paraphrase Crowley, magick is the science and art of causing changes, both in ourselves and our environment, by the exercise of human will. On the face of it, this may seem a very cold, non-spiritual definition of magick. Indeed, many magicians like it that way and would violently disagree with anyone who says that magick has anything to do with humanity's spiritual or religious quest. Magick is, in this sense, a little like Buddhism in that one can be an atheistic or a theistic Buddhist.

However, for me, magick, is very much tied up with spirituality. And paradoxical as it may seem, sexual magick, can be the most spiritual aspect of all magick's many parts - just as it also has the possibility to be its most mechanistic. I like to think that there is a distinction to be made here between 'sexual' magick, which is warm, living and ecstatic with 'sex' magick, which is the very opposite.

This is not to say that all rituals must be sexual rituals, but that in my own practice of magick I am interested in the manifestation of a particular kind of bodily energy; and that it seems to me that a great deal of the magical practice in our long and varied history was based on sexual principles. If this seems too radical I hope to justify my stance in what follows. My plan is roughly as follows: firstly an introductory look at the sexual magick as practised by earlier generations of magicians, during and just before the twentieth century. I used to call this 'old aeon' or 'old style' tantra[1] but perhaps that was arrogant. It is however important to discuss with an impartial and critical eye the works of personalities such as Macgregor Mathers, Edward Berridge, Dion Fortune and the incomparable Aleister Crowley.

Their work was often influenced by the Asian tantrik and Taoist systems of magick. I have therefore often had to venture into that tradition. Dion Fortune said that the 'Eastern way' is not for us 'Europeans'. Well, as Aleister Crowley (1875-1947) quipped, eastern cults, for example Christianity, have always found a fertile home here.

'Tantrik' ideas first reached the West via the collections of British colonials. They were much taken with classics like the *Kama Sutra* and erotic sculpture, often looted from Hindu temples. From this melting pot came some of the late Victorian 'grimoires' such as Randolph's *Magia Sexualis*.

1875 was the year of Crowley's birth and also the foundation of the influential Theosophical Society. The 'TS' was responsible for a fresher infusion of eastern ideas, some of them tantrik, into the western esoteric tradition. Out of the TS came the celebrated Hermetic Order of the Golden Dawn, which used as a magical symbol the Rose Cross, a western form of the tantrik Shri Yantra. Other tantrik concepts and practices were widely used by initiates of the TS and GD. Amongst these we find the use of the tantrik *Tattva (skr:* essence*)* cards and the practice of kundalini yoga. Higher adepts of both these early magical orders practised some kind of sexual magick, itself derived from secret teachers of the then despised tantrik sects.

---

[1] The Sanskrit term 'tantra' has become synonymous with 'sexual magick' in the West and this is undoubtedly a gross simplification. Tantra is the name of a complete magical system, originating in South Asia and incorporating within itself many revolutionary notions about the magical qualities of bodily and sexual forces.

Sexual Magick

Although Crowley often lampooned the Theosophical Society, he included some of Blavatsky's books in the syllabus of his new order the Argentinum Astrum. Crowley at one stage in his magical career styled himself a Buddhist and followed his first magical teacher to Ceylon (Sri Lanka) to pursue this interest. Paradoxically, at the beginning of this century Buddhism had virtually died out in Ceylon, and members of the Theosophical Society played a crucial role in its modern revival there. The style of Buddhism Crowley studied was austere, almost Zen-like (*Skr*: Dhyana). This is reflected in his *Eight Lectures on Yoga*. Yoga, in my opinion, cannot be learned from a book. The student needs to swallow his or her pride and join a good class run by a competent teacher.

A good alternative to yoga is one of the martial arts. An important kind of martial art originated in India and was transformed and syncretised on its eastward journey by Buddhist missionaries of the first few centuries of the common era. The martial arts are full of magical techniques, some derived from tantrism and others from Taoism, the other great influence of modern western magick. The martial arts are especially appropriate for Crowley's magical system Thelema - but at the time he was about, their secrets were even more jealously guarded than those of the sexual gnosis. Karate or Kung Fu certainly cannot be learnt in any meaningful sense without a qualified teacher. When approaching any Eastern technique (or guru) it is as well to keep your wits about you. There are good and bad teachers in all areas of life. There are some, such as the world-famous B K S Iyengar, whose yoga ashram in Poona resembles a medieval torture chamber, full of blocks and ropes, designed to yank your resisting body into the required postures. This kind of training could well lead to injuries if the teacher and indeed the student do not take proper precautions. Sadly, it seems that Crowley was introduced to this kind of yoga training during his stay in India and he in turn passed it on to his students. For instance in Jean Overton Fuller's biography of Victor Neuburg[2], she describes how he found his mouth full of blood after attempting one of Crowley's

---

2 *The Magical Dilemma of Victor Neuburg* (Mandrake of Oxford 1990)

Sexual Magick

exercises in breath control (pranayama). Perhaps we should not be too hard on Crowley, he could only be as good as his teachers. Nowadays there are many competent yoga teachers and one can avoid those who have a tendency to the sadistic. Yoga is about returning the body to its natural rhythm. The body need not be forced into this, it will arise in the course of time if you give the body a chance - the training should facilitate this natural process and no force should be necessary. As Austin Spare put it: 'There is no need for crucifixion.'

Tantra is a magical system that grew out of the yogic practice. Of course there are indications that it is much older than yoga, but the secrets seem to have gone underground for several millennia in India and only began to re-emerge amongst the people who wrote the Yoga Sutras in the first few centuries of the common era.[3] For some obscure reason, some people are apt to think that anything that has survived that long must be without faults. I do not share this view.

Of course, compared to what was going on in the Christian world at the time, India was astonishingly advanced on both a social and political level. Of the many crucial insights made then into the human psyche, the 'rediscovery' of the primal Goddess must rank as amongst the most significant. The Goddess or Shakti became the major source of spiritual power within the Hindu esoteric and magical tradition known as tantrism. However, there was a negative side to this deification of women, who were sometimes worshipped as representatives of the goddess whilst their social status remained inferior. Women were sometimes viewed as instruments in the spiritual advancement of men, especially in the magical or tantrik tradition. These drawbacks should never be forgotten even when working with the undoubtedly effective techniques from this highly creative period of magical history. It is as well to remember that part of being a magician means distinguishing what is good within a tradition and not being afraid to reject what is

---

[3] This is perhaps not the place to argue this point, but one example is the magical power said to reside in the navel chakra as described in the Yoga Sutras at YS III,28.

Sexual Magick

bad. Amongst the things practised by magicians of the past that we must now reject we can of course include, all kinds of blood sacrifice, and all kinds of discrimination, especially against the gender-variant. Throughout this book, I will for ease of writing talk about homosexuality, although I am aware that this is a very narrow term and only gives a partial picture. The homosexual or gender-variant priest and priestess have played a significant role at all times in our long history and this role should be acknowledged and even honoured.[4]

---

[4] Randy Conner, *Blossom of Bone - reclaiming the connections between homoeroticism and the sacred.* (Harper Collins 1993)

Karezza and sexual vampirism

If anyone knows anything about sexual magick it is usually the term *karezza*. The most common meaning amongst occultists of karezza is as the retention of semen. By extension it also means sexual intercourse that lasts a very long time i.e. sexual olympics.

I believe that the origin of this word holds an interesting clue to the technique itself. I take this to be a variant spelling of the Greek word 'corysa' (pronounced koreiza). I hope this is not too fanciful, the information is to be found in the *Oxford English Dictionary* as I try to avoid derivations from Middle Atlantean! 'Corysa' is a runny nose associated with a cold in the head and may well be the equivalent to the Sanskrit 'kasa' or cough. The symbolic thread between the symptoms of a head cold and the delay of orgasm as practised by some occultists may seem impossible to unravel but here is my theory. Crudely put, karezza involves 'sucking' the sexual fluids back into the body. The practitioner may experience this as a physical phenomenon or, more likely, as a psychological or psychical sensation, in which the feelings of the genitals are somehow introverted and draw back up. There are numerous methods of doing this at the moment of orgasm (mulabandha), or holding the breath out of the body and lifting the abdomen up or coughing at the moment of orgasm (One possible experimental method is described below should you want to try it.). Perhaps karezza is a veiled reference to the back pressure in the abdomen that can be created by coughing or other such methods. I should perhaps say that I rarely even bother to try this - because for reasons that may become clear, I think the whole idea is totally flawed.

Most authorities credit **Thomas Lake Harris**[5] with the introduction of the idea if not the term to western aspirants. Thomas

---

[5] T Lake Harris *God's Breath in Man and in Humane Society: Law, Process and Result of Divine Natural Respiration* (Allen 1892); *Wisdom of Angels - Poems* (New York 1857); *The Marriage of Heaven & Earth* (Peace 1903); *The Triumph of Life* (Peace 1903); Anne Taylor L Oliphant (OUP 1982); W P Swainson *Thomas Lake Harris and His Occult Teaching* (Rider 1922); Edward Berridge 'Respiro' *The*

Sexual Magick

Lake Harris (1823-1906) was a Christian Socialist or in his own words, a 'Theo-Socialist'. He was the founder of the Brotherhood of the New life and the Fountain Grove Community in California. He promulgated his own version of the Swedenborgian[6] doctrine that God was both male and female and that every human being, male and female, had a counterpart of the opposite sex. One's duty in life was to find one's counterpart. Harris in the rituals of the Order would hold a [female] member of the brotherhood in his arms, that she might catch a glimpse of her ordained counterpart and the love of Christ would flow down.

> Here find thy mate, forever, two in one
> Circle from star to star, from sun to sun
> In language liquid as the bliss of love
> Repeat below the truth revealed above[7]

Unfortunately for Mrs Thomas Lake Harris, her husband carried this doctrine to extremes. He did not consider that she was actually his particular counterpart and their relationship therefore lacked any physical or emotional fulfilment. One cannot help wondering why he married her in the first place. His biographer thought that this lack of physical contact combined with Harris's notorious philandering contributed towards her early mental breakdown.

Some of the ideas of Thomas Lake Harris, especially those concerning the value of conserving the body's energy in the form of semen and the control of the breath, which was (and still is by some) thought to be the nervous force that causes ejaculation, could well have originated from the Indian tradition. Some of the oldest sexual magick

---

Brotherhood of the New Life, or The Man, The Seer, The Adept, The Avatar, or T Lake Harris, the Inspired Messenger (Allen 1897)

[6] Immanuel Swedenborg (1688-1772), scientist and mystical thinker, the subject of largely 'buried' academic essay by Kant entitled *Dreams of a Spirit Seer*.

[7] *Lyric of the Morning Land* Thomas Lake Harris.

rituals in the world can found within ancient Indian scriptures. Here is such a ritual which I have adapted from an ancient example[8]:

A ritual interlude

Lopamudra [priestess]: For many years I have exhausted myself with abstinence and I have become old just the same. Age wears away the beauty of a body. [Therefore] men should make love to their partners.

The pious sages of ancient times, who conversed about sacred truths with the gods, ceased from abstinence for it did not do any good. [Therefore] women should make love to their partners.

Agastya [priest]: Not in vain is all this (abstinence), which the gods encourage. We two must undertake all struggles. By this we will win the race that is won by a hundred artifices, when we unite together as a pair.

We will reap the rewards of sexual intercourse when we do it in the ritual way. Let us therefore now agree to make love.

(Ritual intercourse now takes place. Then:)

Lopamudra says: Desire for the bull who roars and is held back has overcome me, coming upon me from all sides.

Agastya says: The desire of my swelling phallus which is held back, overwhelms me, coming upon me from all sides.

By this Soma, which I have drunk, in my innermost heart I say: 'Let him forgive us if we have sinned, for a mortal is full of many desires.'

---

[8] Adapted from *Rig Veda* I, 179. Quoted in Wendy Doniger O'Flaherty, *Shiva: the Erotic Ascetic*, (OUP 1973) page 52.

Sexual Magick

Lopamudra is a very interesting woman, a kind of succubus created by the Vedic sage Agastya. The first part of her name (lopa) is probably the name of some variety of bird. After Agastya made her, he brought her up as his daughter until she was old enough (perhaps) for the sexual ritual described above. In the meantime he conquered the demon *Ilvala* to provide her with wealth. Significantly she is said to be the author of the *Rig Veda*, parts of which were written before the ancient Indo-European people moved into the Indian subcontinent from ancient Iran, circa 1500 BCE.[9] Her legend is constantly retold throughout later mythology, especially in connection with Shiva.

It is in the Indian subcontinent that the idea of a spiritual path that was quintessentially sexual was brought to its fullest and most mature version. There is a ritual still practised by tantriks which has five essential ingredients, the so-called five M's (makara) or five powerful enjoyments. This is a kind of love feast in which five things happen or are present in the ritual. These five M's or *makaras* are: meat (mamsa); fish (matsya); alcohol (mada); parched grain (mudra) and sexual intercourse (maithuna).

The five 'Ms', are examples of the 'intentional' or magical language used by tantriks (sandhyâbhâshâ in Sanskrit). The words have a mundane and a secret meaning. The use of this language helps conceal the magician's secrets from the non-initiate but also helps to change the his or her own consciousness towards the desired goal.[10] For example, 'inserting the penis in the vagina, let him not discharge *boddhicitta*.'[11] *Boddhicitta* means 'awakened state of mind', it is also said to mean

---

[9] Information from M Monier-Williams, *Sanskrit-English Dictionary*, New Edition, (OUP 1979)

[10] Earlier translations of this word as 'twilight language' are apparently based on a misspelling. See M Eliade *Yoga, Immortality and Freedom* chapter on 'Intentional Language'; Also A. Bharati. *The Tantric Tradition* (Rider 1970). Although K Zvelebil, who is hardly an inferior scholar, is well aware of Bharati's views but still uses the term 'Twilight language' in his *Siddha Quest For Immortality* (Mandrake 1995).

[11] Shahidullah, *Dohakosha* No. 5 quoted in A Bharati, op cit, page 179.

Sexual Magick

'semen' in tantrik intentional language. The juxtaposition of both meanings in the mind of the magician is very suggestive.

Meat is eaten in spite of the fact that there is a widespread taboo in India against its consumption. Indeed, meat eating is becoming more and more taboo throughout the West. The breaking of taboos seems to play some role in Indian magical practice. Furthermore, the Indian medical system 'science of longevity' (Ayurveda), a discipline closely related to tantrism and magick, tells us that meat and its juices have special pharmacological and psychoactive properties. Perhaps this is what Aleister Crowley was getting at when he recommended that you should eat live food such as oysters or even semen because it had a special energy to it.

Fish could arguably serves a similar function to meat. Fish is very concentrated meat and fulfils an ancient recipe that the 'best meat is the meat of animals that also eat meat'. In India there are also regional variations in what kind of meat it is appropriate to eat. People from the west coast tend to eat more fish (and rice) and this has taken on itself a religious significance. Ignoring these distinctions, is another way of not obeying the rules and also shaking the system up. It must be significant that one of the greatest gurus of the tantrik tradition was named after a fish. His name 'Matsyendranath' may be a reference to the story in which he discovered a great tantrik treatise in the belly of a fish or even perhaps the fact that he was a fisherman and therefore routinely connected with the supposed impurities of that occupation. Such a humble name also suggests a rejection of social class.

However, Alain Daniélou in his crucial study of esoteric Shaivism, *Shiva and Dionysus*[12] maintains that Fish is a code word for urine. The drinking of urine is extremely taboo but also undoubtedly gives the imbiber direct access to many powerful magical and physiological products.[13]

---

[12] Alain Daniélou, *Shiva and Dionysus*, reprinted as *Gods of Love and Ecstasy* by (Inner Traditions 1992)

[13] For more inside information on the use of taboo body products within the magical tradition see: K Zvelebil, *Siddha Quest for Immortality* (Mandrake of Oxford, 1995).

Sexual Magick

In almost every culture you can think of, **Alcohol** is said to have a divine origin - and how right they are. Perhaps because of its ability to loosen up inhibition and the veil between humanity and the gods, it is the substance most often prohibited by many of the world's religions. Given these associations, it should come as no surprise that the iconoclastic sect of tantra put it into the heart of its ritual. The followers of Shiva mix it with ganja or marijuana.[14] In our imaginary ritual we should perhaps extend alchohol to include all ritual drugs. To some religious people, intoxication during ritual is unthinkable. I agree that a room full of totally stoned magicians is not so good, but used with care it has its place.

Sexual Intercourse as a *religious* practice must be the hardest thing to encompass. I have to admit that in all the rituals I have done, this is the least common occurrence. The forces released, whether magical or interpersonal, especially in a group are so difficult to control that symbolic performance seems a safer bet. Sex in a ritual has long been a secret part of humanity's spiritual life. In a recent Australian documentary called *Sacred Sex*, I was particularly struck by the ideas of Annie Sprinkle, who calls herself a 'post-porn modernist'. Although obviously not formally trained in magick she seems to have a natural affinity with it. She has a live stage show that capitalises on her former work as a porn actress, during which she emotionally and sexually challenges all sections of the audience. For example she invites them to come and say hello to her cervix! She also runs encounter-type workshops for women called 'sluts and goddesses' in which she leads people to express their various suppressed personae, both the slutty side and the goddess. In the film she says that she dedicates every orgasm to some concrete result. From the magical point of view this seems a

---

[14] Sanskrit *vijayâ* = (f) 'that which gives victory', bhâng (Hindi); siddhi (Bengali). Earliest mention occurs in *Shatapatha Brâhmana* of 800BCE. According to the Tantriks studied by Bharati, this was an aphrodisiac potion drunk sometime before the taking of the five makaras. In an unconvincing argument, Bharati reasons that it was not included as one of the makaras, because of the time needed for it to work. See Bharati (1970) p. 250.

example we could all follow. At first it may seem mechanical, to make oneself say, I dedicate this orgasm 'to exposing the lies and slanders of the evangelical Christians' but after a while it become automatic and one no-longer has to think too much about it. I find myself instinctively slipping into the magical mind whenever I am lucky enough to have an orgasm these days - which is never enough.

Parched Grain the most obscure of tantra's five powerful enjoyments and in my opinion is a code word for retention of semen. Put another way we can say that parched grain is dried up seed. Traditionally sprouting grains are symbolic of rebirth. In ancient Egypt a tray in the shape of the God Osiris was planted with grain and buried along with other grave goods. The sprouting grain in what Howard Carter called the 'germinating figure of Osiris', was very suggestive of rebirth. Parched grain cannot sprout and thus suggests conservation of energy. In the Buddhist tantrik tradition, mudra is the female partner in the ritual, the 'spiritual support in [the male practitioner's] practice.'[15] Some authorities have suggested that this might also refer to *magnetic* passes or gestures made over the body of a shakti or female priest in order to induce trance. I don't know why the priestess should have all the fun here. However I doubt somehow whether passes made over the body of anyone would induce trance. If someone did that to me I would get very turned on, which is not the same thing as trance at all. Sexual trance, for me, occurs after orgasm in the release phase of the sexual act. Another more obvious interpretation of this symbolism is that 'parched grain' refers to sex 'in itself', rather than sex for procreation. Ridiculous as it may sound, many human societies have developed taboos against recreational sex, and these taboos can only be held in place by quite rigid social conditioning. Any magician worth his or her salt should recognise this and seek to be constantly breaking the taboo.[16]

---

[15] Yeshe Tsogyal, *The Lotus Born - the life story of Padmasambhava* (Shamballa 1993) page 52. This use of the term mudra marks a distinction between Buddhist and Hindu tantrism see A Bharati, *The Tantric Tradition,* (Rider 1970) p. 41

[16] I am grateful to Shantidevi for this insight.

Sexual Magick

However, again following Daniélou it is also quite likely that mudra originally meant specially prepared faecal products of humans and other animals. (See 'fish' above).

From the tantrik and ancient medical (Ayurvedic) point of view, semen is the quintessence of the body's physical components. However above this is a mysterious form of bio-energy called in sanskrit *Ojas*.[17] It strikes me that whatever Ojas is, it is somehow beyond gender and such things as semen, and would make a far better focus for magical transformation. However many yogins seem to prefer to concentrate on their own semen. They try to reverse what they see as an outward flow of energy and thus prolong life and gain immortality. There is still a widespread preoccupation, amongst men from the Indian subcontinent in particular, with semen-loss, and there are well documented reports of young men drinking their own semen after masturbation.[18] The ancient yogis also devised a technique to re-absorb the semen after a, presumably, accidental ejaculation during intercourse. I've also read accounts where the yogi uses his penis as a sucker, helped by his yogically trained muscles, so that he can create a vacuum in his bladder and thus 'hoover up' any potentially wasted sexual fluids. This is the so-called *Vajroli* Mudra or 'Diamond Lock' which must be a variation on the Uddiyana and Nauli Bandhas or locks described in Iyengar's *Light on Yoga*[19].

In brief the technique involves holding the breath after the lungs have been completely emptied of air. Stand up with the back slightly bent, the hands resting gently on thighs. Take a deep breath and then let it out slowly until it is all gone. Now close your mouth, if necessary holding your nostrils closed. This causes a partial vacuum to form in the abdomen and the stomach muscles to be lifted back against the spine. You should be able to help the process by gently lifting up your

---

[17] There is no agreed translation of this word *ojas*, and we are perhaps dealing with a phenomenon not previously noticed in our own tradition.
[18] Charles Leslie (ed) *Asian Medical Systems* (University of California press 1976) page 213.
[19] B K S Iyengar *Light on Yoga* (Allen & Unwin 1968) page 233.

Sexual Magick

abdomen muscles (if you have any) and allowing the vacuum to suck them back toward your backbone. The chin should be kept firmly against the chest to avoid any strain on the heart. You can only maintain this posture for a part of a minute, depending on your fitness, but it should be long enough to begin to sense the flowing upwards of something from the bottommost part of the abdomen. This technique is one that is probably best done with the advice of an expert in order to avoid injury. The subject of Uddiyana recurs below in the context of tantrik geomancy.

The least objectionable use of the above technique is to suppress the sexual currents in order to stop yourself coming too quickly. In my experience, ejaculation occurs when the penis is fully extended at the end of a stroke. If you feel yourself coming too soon and want to delay things then drawing the penis back a little from inside, i.e. sucking it back, can sometimes help. I have spoken to some men who use these techniques to avoid ejaculation during intercourse on a *semi-permanent* basis, although the occasional slip is inevitable. My informants tell me that this is not always pleasant and may even be dangerous as they have experienced a certain amount of pain. Advertisements for instruction in these kind of techniques are surprisingly common if you're really interested.

Anxiety over semen loss leads, in my opinion, to a form of *sexual vampirism*. The more sensitive reader may already have noticed that the focus in much of the above was male and it is he who absorbs the sexual elixir of both partners. Sometimes the esoteric symbolism merely serves to conceal a banal institution of society. I can see in many of these techniques a man taking his pleasure from a woman, and even where he appears the passive male who is served by an active women this is painfully close to the traditional roles of man and wife! An interesting distinction between Buddhist and Hindu tantrism revolves around this point. In Buddhist tantra the male is active and the female represents the principle of quiet wisdom. In Buddhist tantrism the male make a special effort not to ejaculate. In Hindu tantrism, the male

Sexual Magick
represents passive wisdom and the female is the active partner or shakti. In Hindu tantrism the man does eventually ejaculate.[20]

It is very enlightening that the ancient tantriks talked about these nittygritty issues of sex and magical sex in such a frank and revealing way. One essential virtue of tantrik sexual practice is *gentleness*. Gentleness in the sexual act is a direct consequence of the ritual practice. It is very easy for the inexperienced or insensitive male to be too rough and thus ruin things for their partner, this applies both in ritual and mundane intercourse. It is upon this gentle core of traditional tantrik practice that we can recreate a modern sexual magick practice, drawing also on the lessons of the modern way of making love. We need to develop an esoteric sexuality that is based on the experiences of both partners and not just for the benefit of one. Ritual sex, alone, in pairs or groups has its place, along with voyeurism, and many of the techniques described in venerable old tomes like the *Kama Sutra*. But in the end all participants have a right to expect a full and complete experience. Anything less would be to repeat the mistakes of the past. The onesided, vampiric form of sexuality, was in its day an advance on the 'no sex' doctrine of our Victorian ancestors. It did once seem attractive and was secretly taught amongst the higher grades of this century's esoteric orders. We need then to examine this trend in order to understand it and hopefully change it for ever.

Sex and the Hermetic Order of the Golden Dawn

Any study of the western Magical tradition inevitably draws us back to the Hermetic Order of the Golden Dawn. It was formed in 1888 and was active up until the 1920's. There were three basic elements to the Golden Dawn's teaching:

---

[20] See A Bharati, *The Tantric Tradition*, (Rider 1970) p. 41.
K Zvelebil in *Tamil Quest for Immortality* (Mandrake 1995) says that the Tamil Siddhas, who are South Indian Tantriks, also practice conservation of semen, both as a magical technique and as a contraceptive.

Sexual Magick

1. Ceremonial magick
2. The study of Practical Kabbalah
3. Yoga and/or Eastern meditational practices.

The third of these is most relevant here. There is no clear view on the variety of Yoga taught within the Order and it may be that some elements of tantrik yoga were taught in the higher grades. There is a great deal of circumstantial evidence for this, for instance the popularity of the tantrik system of *Tattvas* to represent the elements. 'Tattva' is a sanskrit word which can be translated as 'element'. There are said to be five elements, represented by a yellow or green square for earth, a grey or blue crescent for water; a red upright triangle for fire; a smoky blue or yellow circle for air; and a dark blue or violet ellipse for spirit.

Ithell Colquhoun in *The Sword of Wisdom*,[21] her important biography of MacGregor Mathers, onetime head of the Golden Dawn, advances the theory that he was a practitioner of sexual magick. This is somewhat surprising when one learns that in her letters to Florence Farr, Moina alluded to her own lack of interest in sex; although a wife's lack of interest was not necessarily an inhibition to the average Victorian male. Colquhoun maintains that the couple practised *karezza* during their private experiments in scrying. Moina reputedly sat astride her husband and in this purely ritual intercourse orgasm was avoided. This was, according to Colquhoun, the limit of their sex life, at least with each other, and it was this, she claims, that contributed towards the nervous breakdown of MacGregor Mathers in later life. Many more modern researchers totally reject this above story and it has to be said that Colquhoun, who was for some time a member of Kenneth Grant's Nu-Isis Lodge, would not be the first to have fabricated such stories.

Whatever the facts of his own sexual life, Mathers was particularly protective of fellow Order member Edward Berridge whose psycho-sexual experiments earned him some notoriety. Berridge, who was a disciple of Thomas Lake Harris, popularized the term *karezza*

---

[21] Ithell Colquhoun *The Sword of Wisdom - MacGregor Mathers and The Golden Dawn* (Spearman 1975). The author is an interesting character in her own right. A one-time member of the Surrealist Movement, she was expelled suring its Stalinist phase for her advocacy of magick.

Sexual Magick

and wrote several short pamphlets on Harris's philosophy under the pseudonym Respiro. At one time he was accused of making sexual overtures to the London head of the Golden Dawn, Florence Farr Emery. He was expelled from the Order along with Mathers, Elaine Simpson and Aleister Crowley in 1900 following a protracted power struggle which left Yeats and his circle in control. How much the intricacies of sexual relationships contributed to this is a moot point.

In some senses the poet W B Yeats was a bit of a puritan. For many years of his life he enjoyed the fruits of a spiritual marriage to Maud Gonne, which was, according to contemporary occult gossip, never consummated, physically at least. Yeats says several times in his writings that his libido was the driving force of a great deal of his writing. In later years he felt that the decline of his libido and the waning of his poetic genius were linked. He had had a vasectomy at a time when this operation was a rarity and one must conclude that his reasons were essentially tantrik and that he wanted to conserve what he perceived to be his vital essence. In his sixties he undertook the experimental *Steinach* therapy where desiccated male monkey glands were injected into the muscles. After the death in 1932 of Lady Gregory, one of his closest friends,

> 'his own health went from bad to worse, until he could not climb the stairs without gasping and stopping continually for breath. He might not have had sufficient energy for his last years of work had not a friend half jestingly mentioned to him, early in 1934, the Steinach operation for rejuvenation. . . Yeats was intensely excited and hopeful; to a man who had remade himself over and over during his lifetime, rejuvenation by any means made an intense appeal. In May 1934 a distinguished London surgeon performed the operation, and Yeats almost immediately got a great burst of energy such as he had not had for years.'[22]

It was a fact, well known to ancient physicians, that ingesting the emissions of healthy individuals could alter your own physical and

---

[22] Richard Ellman, *Yeats, The Man and the Masks* (Faber 1961) page 280

psychic balance. Western medicine practices its own sanitised form of tantra, in which patients are given nun's urine, fractions of menstrual blood and other things. Yeats, who knew something of the ancient practice, could have achieved the same result by drinking his guru's semen - if he had the bottle.

Another important personality in our story so far is Dion Fortune. She was a member of the Golden Dawn for a couple of years before her expulsion at the behest of Moina Mathers. Rumour has it that the rift was caused by the publication of Dion Fortune's *The Esoteric Philosophy of Love & Marriage*. An undercurrent of sexual magick and tantra permeates Dion Fortune's entire magical career, the best examples of which are found in her novels, which are scarcely worth reading otherwise. For instance in *The Goat Foot God* the central characters eventually meet at an ancient site of earth energy and invoke the God Pan and his Goddess consort into each other. The consummation of the rite is an act of purest sexual magick.

All of these personalities pale into insignificance, eclipsed by the High Priest of Sexual magick, onetime member of the Golden Dawn, Aleister Crowley. Someone once told me that the essence of Crowley's system, 'is that magick is preparation for making love'. Crowley discovered the full importance of this during a series of magical workings with his lover and fellow magician Victor Neuburg. Sadly,

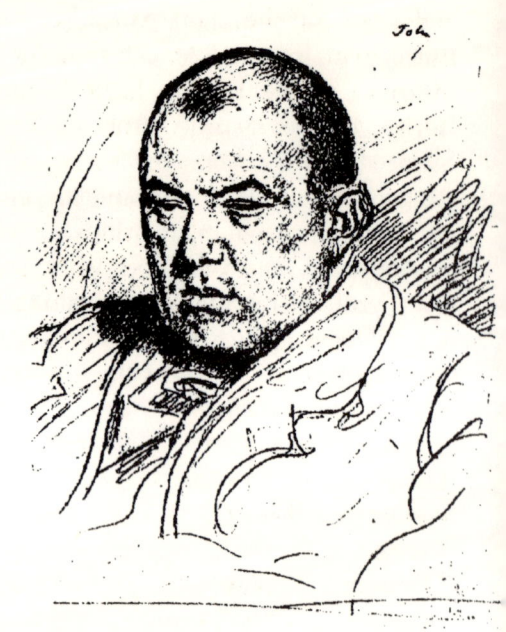

One of many portraits of Crowley drawn by Augustus John (1943: 715).

Sexual Magick

Crowley left very little in the way of instructional material on this important aspect of magical gnosis. And what he did leave is brief and often posed in cryptic language, see for instance *De Arte Magica*. His magical records, with one or two exceptions, are hardly more enlightening. They can be boring in the extreme, with an inordinate amount of space given over to recording what the mage had for breakfast.

It was down to one of his more gifted students of later years, Kenneth Grant, to flesh out the tantrik-sexual gnosis, hinted at in Crowley's writings. Grant added material from more freely available Hindu erotic texts such as the *Ananga Ranga* and the *Kama Sutra*, as well as straight forward tantrik magical texts such as the *Serpent Power*. He drew a whole generation of magicians' attention to a little known type of bodily energy called the Kala - sexual 'rays' that correspond with the waxing and waning moon (see chapter 4). Unfortunately, in some of his writings, Grant, like Crowley, adopts an unpleasant attitude towards the priestess, that often turns genuine seekers away - which is a pity.

However, Grant's fascinating books, especially *Aleister Crowley and the Hidden God*, spurred several magicians of the seventies to ask, 'how can I become a tantrik?' One answer came from 'Dadaji', who knew Crowley in the 1930s, and had been advised by him to go to India to seek enlightenment. Dadaji lived in India from 1953 until his death in 1991. Dadaji had found the horse's mouth and a genuine stream of magical tantra. This he made available to western adepts willing to accept initiation. Some of this material was published in a book entitled *Tantra Magick* (Mandrake *of Oxford* 1990) which has since been republished in India.

However it is undoubtedly Crowley who brought the use of sexual magick to a much more central position in the western esoteric tradition. With the exception of Dion Fortune its use had always been peripheral to ceremonial magick and meditation. Unfortunately Crowley also popularised some of the negative, vampiric aspects of the sexual current. Examples of Crowley's sexual chauvinism are not difficult to find. One of the worst on record must surely be contained in the

Sexual Magick

supposed secret instructions of the ninth degree OTO. In the OTO as reorganised by Crowley, the higher degrees are based upon the use of supposedly secret sexual magical techniques. The eighth degree involved auto-erotic techniques and the ninth degree sexual techniques with a partner of the opposite sex.[23] It is in connection with this that Crowley wrote:

> 'From the duplicity of speech hath sprung infinite confusion in the vulgar mind. For they understand not that man is the guardian of the Life of God, woman but a temporary expedient, a shrine indeed for the God; but not the God.'[24]

It was once put to me that Crowley meant this to be applied equally to men and women, i.e. that 'woman is the guardian of the Life of the Goddess and man is but a temporary expedient.' This is an interesting modern reinterpretation of Crowley's words but personally I doubt if Crowley was proposing such a balanced view. After all he was always very careful in his use of language and if he had meant to talk about Gods and Goddesses would surely have done so. The implication is quite clear that for Crowley the quintessence of the divine was phallic[25], an attitude that reflects the Victorian technique of *karezza* as described earlier. There are still pockets of Thelemites who try to emulate Crowley in these matters, and I read in one recent book that

---

[23] Crowley took the remarkable bold step of introducing an eleventh degree as the counterpart of the heterosexual ninth degree. This eleventh degree was homoerotic. Just by giving this degree the title eleventh, he imbued it with a fantastic status that has worried the more homophobic magicians ever since. For more on this see chapter three 'As brothers fight ye'.

[24] Ed Francis King *The Secret Rituals of the OTO* (Daniel 1973).

[25] This is further made clear by the new rituals Crowley composed for inclusion in his master work *Magick*. For example, the crucial *Liber Samekh* suggests, in coded language, that the magician when projecting his consciousness should visualise it as his own expanding phallus. See also *Star Sapphire* and *Star Ruby*, Crowley's new versions of the old GD Pentagram and Hexagram rituals. Nevertheless, women magicians do use these important rituals although they need a lot of editing.

Sexual Magick

'the western attitude towards sex makes finding a suitable shakti [female partner] a sisyphian task.'[26] This may account for the fact that many women find the Thelemic cult unattractive, at least until they learn how to bend it to their own design.

Despite his shortcomings, Crowley was the medium for a crucial new magical text *Liber Al vel Legis* or the *Book of the Law*, often shortened to *Liber Al* or sometimes just *AL*. This book bears close study and has the rubric of a great deal of sexual magick. In its pages the Thelemic goddess Babalon re-emerges into modern magick for the first time. Babalon[27] has become a new magical archetype for the nineties sexual woman. In the same text, her consort is the Beast, apparently the same as that described in coded form in the *New Testament* book of 'Revelation'. Crowley went to great pains to purge his new magical system from its elements of Christian Kabbalah.[28] So I wonder why he thrust forward these two god-forms which are so quintessentially Christian? I used to think that this was a deliberate act of taboo breaking although now I understand that he was perhaps

---

[26] James Martin, *Sexual Magick in Theory and Practice* (Abraxas 1993)

[27] The paradox is that a chauvinist like Crowley should be the vehicle for such a liberating female archetype. However a contemporary priestess of Babalon, currently working with the GDS says that she finds the work of Jack Parsons on Babalon of far greater value to the modern practitioner.

[28] For those who doubt this consider the original Pentagram rite as published, amongst other places, in Crowley's book *Magick*. The ritual is still central to much Hermetic magick, including my own. In this ritual one invokes the four elemental angels, and uses the elemental variations on the tetragrammaton. The beginning of the kabbalistic cross is virtually identical with the last lines of the, admittedly ancient, *Lord's Prayer*. The final banishing is often accomplished by vibrating the five-fold name of god which I will only render here as Jesus. Later on in *Magick*, Crowley published his revised versions of the pentagram and hexagram rituals, with symbolism more in keeping with the thelemic system. He called these rituals the Star Ruby and the Star Sapphire.

Sexual Magick

referring to a secret kabbalistic commentary.[29] Babalon[30] the whore, the Great Beast[31] and the androgyne Baphomet are in reality modern magical archetypes and have very little in common with any known mythology of the ancient world.

Crowley claimed that *Liber Al* was dictated to him by a preternatural intelligence over a period of three days in April 1904. Whatever its origins, its contents came to dominate his magical work from then on. Many view *Liber Al* as almost akin to a new tantra, in the sense that it combines the form and content of a tantrik text with the characteristics of a western grimoire.

Ritual magick, including the Thelemic variety, so-called because of the importance in *Liber Al* of the Greek concept Thelema or [free] Will, tends to categorise various kinds of magical work according to the eleven spheres or degrees of the Kabbalistic Tree of Life. There are thus said to be three varieties of sexual magick, corresponding to the eighth, ninth and eleventh spheres on the tree of life. Personally I think this categorisation is obsolete as I hope to explain below. However, before doing so, I'd best rehearse the supposed differences. The eighth sphere is usually taken to be sexual magick of an auto-erotic kind and the ninth sphere refers to sexual magick of a heterosexual variety. Crowley

---

[29] Like many magicians I have been inoculated by fundamentalist Christianity from ever looking at this book, but when I did force myself to I was very struck by verse 4: 'to the seven churches that are in Asia' which could read 'To the seven palaces that are in Assiah'.

[30] Crowley 'corrected' the spelling of this word using magical principles. The ancient city state was and is spelt Babylon. The 'whore of Babylon' as written about in the *New Testament, Book of Revelation*. If John of Patmos had given her name it may well have been Inanna. Crowley 'corrected' the spelling to Babalon, numerical value 156, as heralded in his own book of revelation - *Liber Al*. This is new name of an ancient feminine force. I must at this point acknowledge Jake Stratton-Kent, an expert on English kabbalah, whose talk at the Eighth National Symposium of Thelemic Magick on *Christianity and Thelema*, first got me thinking about these issues.

[31] Some ancient authorities give the beast of revelation the numeration 616 as well as 666. See *Bible*, RSV version.

Sexual Magick

worked with a version of the Tree of Life that had an additional or eleventh sphere, sometimes called by more traditional Kabbalists a 'false' sephira. Far from viewing this eleventh sphere as false, Crowley's mystical text *Liber Al* viewed it as *the* magical sphere. Once again, Crowley is moving magick away from Christian kabbalistic roots toward a more tantrik and taboo breaking form. 'My number is 11,' it says in *Liber Al*, 'as are their numbers who are of us.'[32] Crowley reasoned that the magick most appropriate to the eleventh sphere, or to give it its Hebrew name *Daath*, would involve some kind of reversal of the practices of the ninth degree. For some magicians the idea of working with the sphere of Daath is anathema because of its association with evil. However Daath in Hebrew translates as 'knowledge',[33] which makes it a worthy focus for the magical quest. The kind of reversal practised by Crowley was homosexual magick or more specifically a magical technique involving anal intercourse which he called 'through the unmentionable vessel' (*pvn--per vas nefandum*).

There are of course several good reasons why Crowley chose this path, not least of which must have been his own bisexuality, which is openly discussed in the *Confessions*. Homosexual techniques have an anti-social element and therefore psychological 'power' or edge and this is parallel to the ideas behind many tantrik and magical rituals which play upon the reversal of the commonplace behaviour and morality. Thus the eating of meat in a vegetarian community can have the same liberating effect as anal intercourse in a sexually inhibited straight society. It was this anti-social current that Crowley found so good at producing magical consciousness or what we might call the magical

---

[32] Al I. 60

[33] *Kabbalah* Gershom Scholem (New American Library 1974). Scholem's books are a bit dry but give some essential source material. He was very hostile to the magical tradition and claimed that magick was a peripheral or degenerate aspect of the early 'merkavah' mysticism. This interpretation has recently been seriously challenged in a lecture by Peter Schäfer, published as: *Gershom Scholem Reconsidered: the aim and purpose of early Jewish Mysticism*, published by the Oxford Centre for Postgraduate Hebrew Studies 1986.

Sexual Magick

mind. A final and by no means trivial reason for adopting this technique is to be found in the history of homo-erotic magick, which contains rituals and magical formulae of great power; something discussed further below.

Of course, homo-erotic magick is not the only way to introduce elements of reversal or perversity into your magick. I have already commented upon a group of magical texts with many similarities to Crowley's *Liber Al*. These are the tantras, from whose perspective the same effect is realized by heterosexual intercourse, which is widely considered to bring contact with taboo substances such as semen, sexual fluids and menstrual blood.

Menstruation can also be associated with the so-called false sephira or sphere of Daath on the Tree of Life. One reason why Daath has in the past been labelled 'evil' may have something to do with its periodic or temporary manifestation. The possibility of its having an illusionary nature makes it a natural alternative symbol on the Tree of Life to the Lunar or Yesodic sphere as a symbol of menstruation. One difference between Yesod and Daath is that in the sphere of the moon illusions are created whereas in the sphere of Daath they are destroyed, which is one possible definition of knowledge.

Sexual intercourse during menstruation is viewed in many cultures as dirty, defiling and taboo. From a magical point of view intercourse during inappropriate times and with matter that is 'out of place' is looked at as something with great creative and magical potential. From the classical tantrik point of view, the dark lunar current present at menstruation is, under certain circumstances, arguably the most powerful magical emanation available. This in reflected in the words of *Liber Al* as 'The best blood is of the moon - monthly.' Menstruation is often used as a symbol for esoteric events for instance the opening of the third eye or the movement of the body's bio-energy or Kundalini to the Ajña Chakra.

The Magical and mundane potential of menstruation has been described at length in an important book by Penelope Shuttle and Peter Redgrove, *The Wise Wound - Menstruation & Everywoman* (first published in 1978). The authors claim that many women experience

Sexual Magick

two peaks of sexual desire in the course of a monthly cycle. These peaks correspond to ovulation and menstruation. Although this is a rather schematic approach to sexual desire they do manage to draw some interesting conclusions. On a biological level the first of these peaks may well correspond with the time when intercourse is most likely to lead to conception. In the world constructed for us by the patriarchal religions, the second peak has no such function and is often either ignored or despised. However Redgrove and Shuttle believe that the peak at menstruation also has a function, although this time of a metaphysical kind. Furthermore they speculate that it is the subconscious knowledge of the creative potential of sex during menstruation that leads to a conflict between nature and society. And this in turn results in guilt and maybe, according to the authors, pre-menstrual tension. However from a magical perspective it is this second peak of sexual desire at menstruation that is treasured, along with those other occasions when this is possible, for its ability to engender another variety of offspring, the inner or magical child. The 'child' in this context is seen as a kind of 'thought-form', creative act or urge that is able to take on an astral life of its own. Alternatively it can be seen as a symbol of human consciousness reborn and transformed to its true potential.

Three spirits in a chamber

I said earlier that I thought the idea of three kinds or grades of sexual magick was obsolete. Indeed I think there is just sexual magick. There seems to me no *essential* difference between the sexual magick that occurs between heterosexual or homosexual partners. I doubt if there is any essential difference between sexual magick occurring at the time of menstruation or at other special times, or if there is a difference it is merely one of degree or intensity. And furthermore, I see auto-erotic magick in the same light. My saying this also serves to remove some of the stigma that still attaches itself to some kinds of sexual magick, especially the auto-erotic variety.

As if to underline this I now intend to take as a possible example of sexual magick a ritual that on the face of it appears to be auto-erotic

Sexual Magick

- but is it? My example is taken from a very rare manuscript that resides in the Bodleian Library, Oxford. All the basic ingredients are here.

> 'A treatise on the conjuration of Angels with experiments in crystal and directions for fumigations.'

This manuscript is now in the Bodleian Library. It is the work of Moses Long the conjuror (1683) of Gloucester. The manuscript was bought by Rawlinson from Thomas Herne who had it in 1731. Herne thought it a transcript of a sixteenth century manuscript from the collection of Allen, a conjuror who lived at Shifford near Bampton in Oxfordshire; before that it was in the possession of several other 'cunning' men, including Cornelius of Oxford and Seckford, a glover of Oxford.

Much of the text is therefore contemporary with John Dee's spiritual diaries and shows the extent of occult experimentation in the sixteenth century.

....

An Experiment for three Spirits done in a chamber three nights

A true experiment proved in Cambridge, Anno 1557 of three spirits to be done in a chamber, whose names are Durus, Artus and Aebeddell.

....

Rise early on the first moonday after the new moon and in the hour of the moon cut three rods. The stock or body of a palm tree and not on the top, with a new, sharp knife, never used. On the knife let be written on the blade:

+ Alpha + on one side and

Sexual Magick

+ Omega + on the other

With this knife in thy hand say

'In the name of god the father I have sought thee rods', so taking hold of them saying 'in the name of god the son, I have found you rods' saying

'In the name of the holy ghost I cut you all three'.[34]

Then take fine parchment and cut three pieces and on the first piece write Duxus [sic], on the second write Artus and on the third write Aebeddell. Then first take the name Durus and wrap it about one of the rods and so do the rest in order. Then take the first rod or wand in thy hand and say:

'through the blessed power and mercy of god, I command thee rod, by virtue of the rod wherewith the prophet Elias[35] raised upon the waters between him and Eliseus, that ye spirit, whose whole name is written and wrapped about thee, be obedient to me, always, whensoever I shall call him. Then set down the rod in the east end of the chamber. [in another hand: Therefore because I know not whether they be good or evil, I advise you not to meddle with them, as I have advised in others so in these]

Then take the second rod in thy hand saying:

---

[34] The use of Christian concepts freely interlaced with hermetic ones is a feature of the magick of this period. If you don't like it you could try reminding yourself that many of these traditional prayers are very ancient indeed and like the psalms, widely used in magick, they can be traced back to Egyptian and Sumerian sources of magick. If you're still not convinced try substituting your own prayer but be careful to preserve the threefold symmetry that permeates the whole ritual.

[35] Elijah, see obscure account of this miraculous happening in the presence of his successor Elisha or Eliseus in *Bible* 2 Kings 8.

Sexual Magick

'Oh ye rod or wand through the blessed power and mercy of god, I command thee by virtue of the rod wherewith Moses turned the waters of Egypt into cloud that the spirit whose name is written and wrapped about thee be obedient unto me whensoever I call him. '

Then set down in the west part of the chamber.

Then take the third rod in thy hand saying:

'Oh ye rod or wand through the blessed power and mercy of god I command thee, by that virtue, might and strength of the rod wherewith the Holy Angel measured the temple of god, that the spirit whose name is written and wrapped about thee, be obedient and true to me whensoever I call him.'

Then set it down in the south of they chamber and say as follows:

[There then follows a long exhortation which may not be to the modern taste, but in terms of the techniques of the sixteenth century is likely to have been very effective. Jan Fries in his book *Visual Magick* describes a little the modern equivalent of slow prayer as a powerful way of invoking the magical mind.
The heavy Judeo-Christian flavour of this section should not lead the reader to doubt that the writer was every bit a magician as you or I. Magick, like shamanism, is not a religion, but a state of mind, that is equally at home in any given religious context. Perhaps that is why, when religions come and go, magick has been and always will be here.]

Then 'I require and command you sprits all three, in the name of god the father, son and Holy ghost, that as you dread and owe obedience unto the true, omnipotent and undoubtedly god who hath created the universal world and all creatures and hosts of heaven and earth and through his infinite omnipotent power and virtue in

Sexual Magick

all hierarchies of Angels and intellectual and spiritual and celestial and elemental creatures and all effable and ineffable names and powers of god and works of the glorious true, incomprehensible good and merciful god, that as + Jesus Christ is the son of the living god and was conceived by the holy ghost and borne of the virgin Mary and suffered in the flesh upon the cross, for all believing penitent sinners and rose again on the third day and is ascended up into heaven sitting at the right hand of god the father for all believing and repentant sinners and for true as he is + Alpha and Omega + and shall come to judge the quick and the dead and the world with fire, that so true and certainly that these three spirits, Durus, Artus and Aebeddell be obedient and appear visible in this chamber and whensover I shall at any time call ye in the name of god the father, son and holy ghost through virtue, power and obedience due to the glorious Lord + Jesus Christ + at whose name the knees of things in heaven and things in earth and things under the earth so bow, so be it done through the might power and virtue of + Jesus Christ + Fiate Fiat Amen,[36] ever as you will answer your obedience to these powers and virtues at the dreadful day of judgement.

[Now comes the point stated so briefly you could almost miss it, as I did the first time I read it:]

'So come ye gently and peaceably in the form and shape of three beautiful ladies and truly to answer *all* [sic] my will and desire in all before said.

In nomine patris filius et spiritus sancti, Amen fiat amen.

---

[36] An example of what Crowley called 'barbarous' names or the magical voice (voce magicae), words of power to be vibrated by the magician.

This must be done three nights and [on] the third night three spirits will appear to thee at thy *bedside* and will ask what is thy will and desire. Then say 'welcome ye fair and gentle spirits whom god hath created.'

Then say - 'I charge and command you upon your obedience to that Lord god by whose power you are sent hither that you truly tell me the truth of all my requests and demands without any lying or deceit or delays, now present and all times, when and whensoever I shall call you in the name of the father, son and holy ghost. *Three forms and one god,* to whom be all glory, honour, might, majesty and dominion ascribed without end. Amen'

The Licence To Depart[37]

Then having answered thy demands say - 'in the name of god the father, son and holy ghost I command you to depart in peace to the place god hath appointed you, not hurting me nor any creature under heaven and being ready when I shall call you again as before said - Amen.'

A exhortation follows in which the 'Artist' is warned of the dangers of traffic with spirits. Through techniques like this the magician creates spirits that commune with him or indeed her most probably via lucid dreams. The ritual seems to begin with formal invocation but the result comes when the magician or 'artist' is in his bed and probably asleep. A modern magician would probably help things along a bit by masturbating a little or even to orgasm before sleeping. Alternatively two (or perhaps more) magicians might 'incubate' the spirit dream by having sex before sleep. In either of these scenarios, it is my view that

---

[37] Never omitted in these kinds of potentially dangerous magick. Such formulae are traditional and still widely in use. They are undoubtedly very old indeed and help prevent the Faustus complex.

Sexual Magick

the distinction between auto-erotic, homosexual and heterosexual magick is so blurred as to be meaningless.

The only important thing is that a special type of dream is incubated during which the spirits invoked visit the magician or magicians in sleep. Alternatively, the vision manifests during the trance induced by a good sex session. In either case, this is an important method of magical experimentation, one that I know works and which can have profound and far-reaching results.

I have also found that the experience works well the other way round. The formal part of the ritual is done in the evening, perhaps a version of the example given. The spirits or spirit invoked in the ritual returns in a more sentient form during sleep. Sometimes the result is an orgasm or several orgasms during sleep. But more often than not, sleep is constantly interrupted and the night is one long session of karezza. In the morning I record the words and events that happened during the night visions. I have sometimes been literally aching with lust by this time and am grateful for the opportunity to earth the energy with a pleasant sex session. The body feelings are not unpleasant but they can be a bit overwhelming. However they will subside after an hour or so.

Things can also go wrong so it is wise to take precautions. If you already have problems distinguishing between the real and the astral world then perhaps you had best try another technique. If you think you might find it hard to banish the spirits when you've had enough and worry about the consequences, then once again, this is a good reason to try something else.

Auto-erotic fantasies during sleep fulfil all the conditions of sexual magick. The encounter is very real and often ends with a wonderful orgasm. These astral encounters are very real and profound and I certainly count mine as some of miy most significant magical experiences - although strictly speaking the dividing line between this and masturbation is difficult to draw. (More on sexual experience in chapter 4).

Homosexuality

Homosexuality has a long and ancient association with the magical tradition. Even so it is rare for magicians to express anything other than derision for homosexuals and homosexuality. The magical literature abounds in attitudes that can only be described as *homophobic*. Magicians may have radical, sometimes even revolutionary ideas in many things, but almost always adopt the reactionary views of the ruling orthodoxy in this matter. It is important to unravel this mental knot, if we are ever to hope to reach a balanced approach to the substance of sexual magick.

In many ways we are fortunate in having Aleister Crowley as a role model, for he appears to have had a homosexual love affair whilst still at university and was a life-long bisexual, even weaving his bisexuality into a magical system (more on this in chapter three). In the *Confessions*[38] he writes about his earliest homosexual affair with a fellow Cambridge student:

> 'The relation between us was the ideal intimacy which the Greeks considered the greatest glory of manhood and the most precious prize of life. It says much for the moral state of England that such ideas are connected in the minds of practically everyone with physical passion.'

Despite this, in later years he was to regard homosexuality, when not part of a magical ritual, in the words of the *Bible* 'as an abomination'[39]. One cannot help wondering if there is not an element of pose not to say hypocrisy in this statement.

Another 'great' occultist of the twentieth century was Dion Fortune. Her views on this subject are especially disappointing as she was widely considered to be a liberal and a progressive. Writing in the 1930s:

---

[38] *The Confessions of Aleister Crowley - An Autohagiography* edited by John Symonds and Kenneth Grant (London, Cape 1969) page 142.
[39] Aleister Crowley *Magick* (RKP 1972) page 165.

Sexual Magick

'An unnatural vice known as homosexuality, the offence for which Oscar Wilde received a sentence of imprisonment. It is a very cruel form of vice, as the victims are usually boys and youths on the threshold of life. It is also very infectious, spreading in an ever widening circle as those who have become habituated to it in their turn proselytise for victims.The many supporters of these people defend them by asking how it can be that men of such dedicated lives, who give such lofty and beautiful teaching can be addicted to such foul practices. For those who have made a serious study of occultism the explanation is self-evident. It was this particular vice which was one of the chief causes of the decadence of the Greek Mysteries.'[40].

One may perhaps be inclined to forgive this kind of things coming from the Edwardians; perhaps they knew no better. However one wonders why Dion Fortune had never encountered the pioneering ideas of sexologist Magnus Hirschfeld or Havelock Ellis?[41] With depressing regularity Dion Fortune's absurd ideas on sexuality recur in successive modern works on magick. It would be laughable if it were not so sad. For example:

---

40 Dion Fortune *Sane Occultism* (Aquarian Press 1987) page 83. Actually her ideas on many other areas of occultism are becoming increasingly untenable. See my remarks made in the introduction on her 'ethnocentric' approach to magick with talk of 'race dharma' and similar non-sense. On an occult level she is hardly a brilliant authority for example in her 'standard' text, the *Mystical Qabalah*, she makes the most puerile comments about the origins of the rosy cross. Crowley people sometimes tolerate her because of her supposed secret affiliation with the man, but apparently even this has been exaggerated to say the least. I do however agree with this statement from *Internet Kabbalah FAQ*: 'The *Mystical Qabalah* [was] one of the first books to relate the sephirotic tree to everyday experience and for this reason it is a useful beginner's book.'
41 Charlotte Wolff *Magnus Hirschfeld - A Portrait of A Pioneer in Sexology* (Quartet 1986).

Sexual Magick

'Another common form of deviation is linked with the differentiation of the sexes. One sees men refusing to be men and women refusing to be women. This does not refer only to the more obvious forms of perversion such as homosexuality, but also to the quite common manifestation of "cocksure women and hen-sure men" as D H Lawrence described it.'

This is from Gareth Knight a self-styled authority on 'white magick'.[42] In the same book the author discusses the question of sexual polarity in relation to the sphere of Netzach on the Tree of Life and this is what he says:

'On its more intense levels it can be dangerous with undedicated people for, by a confusion of the planes a high powered mutual stimulation on the mental and higher emotional levels can degenerate into homosexuality. In spite of the modern spate of apologetics for this form of lower emotional and physical relationship, it is a perversion and evil. It is perhaps as well to state this quite categorically as it is a form of vice likely to be on the increase with the lesser differentiation in physical sexual characteristics of the Aquarian type of human now coming into the world. This increasing lack of differentiation is becoming quite common; there are increasingly few men nowadays who could grow a really patriarchal beard and women, from the buxom mammalians of classical painting are becoming more boyish and angular in figure, to say nothing of the occasional much publicized actual changes from one sex to another. Homosexuality, like the use of drugs, is one of the techniques of black magick.[43]

---

42   Gareth Knight *A Practical Guide to Qabalistic Symbolism* (Helios 1976) Vol II page 56.
In the 1980s Gareth Knight was still peddling the same line and is quoted in Tanya Luhrman's *Persuasions of the Witch's Craft* as saying that no real magician could be homosexual.

43   *op cit* Vol I page 156.

Sexual Magick

Surely this is one magical book we should consign to the flames? Apart from commenting on the appalling ignorance of western symbolism and mythology displayed by these passages, all I can add is that if Gareth Knight represents 'white magick' I know which side I'm on! The next two chapters will examine a little more deeply some of this ancient symbolism. It won't have escaped attention that the above passages refer to male homosexuality and therefore reflect the traditional invisibility of the lesbian. In Nik Douglas and Penny Slinger's book *Sexual Secrets* the authors say that they have no *objection* to lesbianism as long as it is used as a supplement to heterosexuality and not as an alternative. It is sad to see an otherwise brilliant book marred by this kind of ill-informed prejudice. Their attitude towards male homosexuality, which is completely rubbished, is even worse. It is a shame that they attempt to justify their hang-ups by recourse to the more puritanical threads that run through some tantrik sources. [44]

The magical importance of homosexuality

In tantrik magick the Sanskrit term 'kantâ' is often used and this denotes 'the beloved'. Flowing from this is an important tenet of sexual magick that one's partner, physical or astral, should be loved. Love is a phenomenon equally well manifested between homosexuals as well as heterosexuals or for that matter any of the other genders. (I shall in fact describe in chapter three a little of the idea that there are more than two genders and that this idea lies behind a great deal of important magical symbolism.) Love is always missed out of a great deal of pseudo-occult theorizing concerning homosexual sex magick. It is an undoubted fact that two men or two women can love each other with the same intensity and authenticity as any other couple. This is often the starting point of genuine magical work and not merely some purely accidental physical aspects of the sexual act itself. The power of *Love under Will* is said by some to be able to transform the physical secretions of the body into magical elixirs in an unparalleled manner. For others pure lust, i.e. a

---

44   Nik Douglas & Penny Slinger *Sexual Secrets* (Arrow 1979).

Sexual Magick

driving desire for sexual gratification, may accomplish the same results, although personally I feel that the idea of love encompasses physical desire and therefore has a more transcendental quality.

Sexual magick today

This must be the right place to set out some possible experimental directions for sexual magick as we approach the new millennium. Paradoxically sexual magick implies a duality of two or more partners and yet is often said to have as its ultimate aim the dissolution of this distinction. Personally I believe that there are two basic principles in our universe and no further reduction is possible. These two basic principles are sometimes called spirit and matter. In ancient mythologies these two principles were often symbolized either as male and female or as twins. The dualistic philosophy of sexual magick is at odds with other more pessimistic and austere creeds. Existence is for us is in the words of *Liber Al* 'pure joy'. Of course describing the two principles is one thing, disentangling their relationship with each other is another. In fact the way spirit and matter interact has been the object of humanity's spiritual quest since at least the beginning of historical time. As part of this quest we should be mindful of the hermetic dictum 'As above, so below' which surely means that we hold within our own physical bodies the entire secrets of the universe if we could but see it. Modern students of alchemy have drawn attention to the exceptional parallel between Indian and Hermetic sources.[45] One of the clearest comes from an ancient Indian medical text where the author Charaka says: 'The wise know this to be true: that the individual is a microcosm of the universe. All material and spiritual phenomena ... are present in the individual. Similarly all those present in the individual are also contained in the universe.'[46] There has been much talk of magical elixirs, holy grails and

---

[45] Michael L Walter 'The Role of Alchemy and Medicine in Indo-Tibetan Tantrism' PhD Diss. 1980 (University of Indiana, Bloomington)

[46] *Charaka Samhita*, section on embryology, English translation by Sharma and Dash, (Chowkhamba 1977) p. 393 (CS. Nidanasthana IV).

Sexual Magick

philosophers' stones. Surely these things must in some sense exist within our own bodies?

In my opinion the obscure language of the alchemists refers to a process occurring within the body and to the repercussions of this within our own consciousness. This is not the place to write a history of western alchemy, but it may have escaped the notice of western scholars that there is a direct link between tantrik ideas and the western tradition of alchemy. Sometimes when I read the works of Thomas Vaughan, the English Renaissance alchemist, I feel sure he is actually quoting from an Indian source. In the Indian alchemical tradition, which is to all intents and purposes the same thing as the tantrik tradition, the term 'rasa' is used to denote metallic mercury. However originally this crucial magical concept, rasa, was always used to describe the transcendental fluids of the human body.

Rasa has been called the 'substance of lust'. Like all interesting Indo-European concepts it is both a physical and a metaphysical thing. Rasa could denote any of the bodily fluids, and especially those secreted when the body is sexually aroused. It also refers to the emotional or aesthetic sentiment that is part of the act of love. Rasa is also used to refer to the sentiments that can be evoked by music and the arts. Medieval alchemists talk of a 'first matter' which by a series of mystical transubstantiations is somehow transformed into a magical substance, which for them was represented by gold or the philosopher's stone. Ancient information from the tantrik roots of alchemy led me to conclude that the 'first matter' of the alchemists is another name for this highly novel concept 'rasa'. It was therefore intimately connected by them with the sexual act and its consequent sexual secretions. There is no doubt that Thomas Vaughan actually experimented on his own semen. Sex would have been seen as an odd thing for an intelligent man in Tudor England to be experimenting with, and this may account for the notion that something universally despised was transformed into something glorious. 'Despised' is perhaps too literal, but certainly not valued in a spiritual or magical sense. Thus lead becomes gold and an ordinary human consciousness become super-conscious.

Sexual Magick

The sexual act is only likened to lead because it can result in physical offspring. The same act has an entirely different effect if infused with a magical intent, when, in the words of *Liber Al*, it falls under the influence of 'Love under Will'. The first and perhaps most significant step in this process is to make a conscious decision to view your sexuality as something magical and allow all things to reinforce this intention. Thus any sexual act is also a magical ritual.

Magical partners should regularly make a dedication to each other within the sacred space of the circle. A partner's cunt, penis, or whatever, can be worshipped as the visible representation of the divine. Some people may find that they have a mental block against visualising a deity presiding over the genitals. This may well be a hangover from your previous conditioning, perhaps by one of the religions 'of the book'. One of the tasks of any magician is to try to identify the unconscious taboos and sources of guilt within his or her consciousness and to remove them. Understanding the esoteric doctrine of the body is part of this process of deconditioning. So for instance you should know that when two bodies are joined in a sexual act they replicate the cosmos in its primeval or unevolved state.

You need to replace the old mythology that you have unconsciously absorbed during your childhood with more authentic or fresher myths from the magical tradition. For example the ancient Indian myth of creation that compares the process to the churning of the ocean of milk by the gods. The ocean is churned by Shiva who takes on the form of a phallic and cosmic mountain. Coiled about this mountain is a gigantic serpent and the Gods facilitate the act of creation by hauling on the ends of the serpent thus causing the mountain to churn the ocean. Out of the churning of the ocean countless elixirs *and poisons* are produced.[47] This is only one example of many other highly charged and sensual myths. Such images can be enacted or called to mind during an act of sex or sexual magick. The churning of the cosmic

---

[47] Wendy D O'Flaherty *Hindu Myths* (Penguin 1975).

waters leads to orgasm[48]. Before and after orgasm several bodily secretions and ejaculations are produced by *both* partners. It is my belief that they are transformed from their normal state by whatever was going on in your mind during their production. Thus if you have magick on your mind this will effect the secretions. If you have just spent the whole night communing with Babalon on a spirit level as a result of dream incubation, then this will be concatenated into the sex fluids. We tend to view them as lifeless and fit only for rapid disposal, but in fact they bear minute (perhaps homoeopathic) fractions of some

---

[48] The modern Hermetic tradition, heavily under the influence of sexologists such as Wilhelm Reich, has developed its own special kind of sexual magick. Some of the modern accounts of Taoist body magick seem to place an inordinate amount of stress on avoiding orgasm altogether. This may well be a distortion of the original doctrine. For example accounts of Taoist masters, usually of advancing years, who claim to have intercourse several times a day but never to ejaculate should not be taken at face value. My research leads me to suppose that there is a big difference in the quality of their sexual experience. One of my informants rather dismissively called this 'old man's sex'. There is plainly a conflict here. Modern society places a great deal of value on the kind of peak physical performance that can be obtained in youth. Taoist philosophy seems to want to avoid peaks and troughs, finding instead a kind of median way that persists throughout life. I have certainly met martial artists who in their late thirties feel 'over the top' and regret they do not have the edge they once possessed in their early twenties. The Taoists are surely have a point when they say this is not a useful life philosophy and that if people must think in terms of peaks, why not sixty years of age, half the ideal Taoist life span? By western standards I am in decline although I don't feel it. It makes sense for me to adopt the Taoist approach, although only time will tell whether I am deluding myself. Sex, as I get older, may become a much slower and less urgent process. Whether or nor this makes it better or 'more spiritual' is still, for me, a moot point. As the saying goes: 'we are different and therefore equal'. For all stages of life, sexual encounters should, so I believe, be fulfilling and complete bodily experiences that induce a post-orgasmic trance. It follows from this that falling asleep after sex is not necessarily as bad as some supposed 'experts' would maintain.

Sexual Magick

of the most important and at the same time, mysterious substances the body can produce. This is one meaning of the 'strange drugs'[49] taken by the magician. The sexual magician should allow some time for these to be re-absorbed as they are said to be able to change your consciousness and your body.[50]

One would like to think that this type of energy could be released in a group. This would have to be a very intimate affair and necessarily restricted in numbers. I suspect that this is rarely if ever the way things work in the dwindling tantrik groups of the Indian sub-continent. It would be so easy for it to degenerate into a rather unsatisfactory orgy. It may take years before western groups are ready for this kind of practice. In wiccan groups one often hears the phrase that participation requires 'perfect love and perfect trust,' and this does indeed seem a necessary part of sexual magick. Modern wiccans also use a term 'skyclad', a translation from the Sanskrit *digambari* 'clothed in space' reputedly as a visible sign of this trust and vulnerability.

One intermediate point between sexual magick in pairs and in groups might be found in the cult of the Sahajiyas.[51] This is a cult, with many similarities to tantrism, although it is based on the mythology of Krishna, the dark tribal incarnation of Vishnu, and Radha, the wife of a herdsman, but also Krishna's ritual partner. This pattern is mirrored in the Sahajiya ritual group, a truly eternal triangle. The women initiates of the cult form temporary relationships with male initiates other than their husbands. Between these two an important relationship develops through which they come to experience the rasa or true religious love for the divine, which they see in each other. The driving forces for the growth of this rasa is the unconsummated love between them. In some

---

[49] See *Liber Al*
[50] Peter Redgrove says in the *Black Goddess and the Sixth Sense* that they should not be allowed to come into contact with the air, as they lose their potency.
[51] My attention was first drawn to this topic by an article in the first and second issues of *Starfire*, although the standard sources are Bose, *Sahajiya Cult*, Dasgupta's *Obscure Religious Cults* and Dimock, *The Secret Moon*. E Dimock, *The Hidden Moon*, (Rider).

Sexual Magick

cases ritual intercourse does take place, but it is quite possible to enter this magical relationship solely on an astral or non physical level. These magical alliances may end at any time, and it is the elements of fantasy, unrequited love and the unattainable that can give it a power to create physical rasa in a similar way to the 'three spirits in a chamber ritual' described earlier.

For us sensitive types, vulnerability and being naked is a privilege that can only be enjoyed with those we love, otherwise one runs the risk of merely adopting another mask. Perhaps this is why most practitioners of this magick work with one partner or within one group over a number of years. There are many other conditions that need to be met before sexual magick can be widely practised in groups. For example the traditional roles and power relationships forced on magical groups by previous generations need to be changed. Central to this is the desire for a complete balance and equality between the various participants, whatever their gender. The primary and innocent state of bliss as sometimes represented in the kabbalistic tradition as the Garden of Eden before the fall is the ultimate destination of the magical quest. I hope to see you there some day soon.

Chapter 2
Serpent Power[1]

Body techniques may well be necessary conditions for the attainment of certain mystical states. This chapter concerns some of this body magick.[2] No one who is sexually active can doubt the fact that

---

[1] (A background paper prepared for the second National Symposium of Thelemic Magick, 24th October 1987 ev.)

[2] Marcel Mauss (1979) 'Body Techniques' in *Sociology and Psychology - Essays* (RKP: London) pp. 95-123

This is a reprint of Mauss's groundbreaking essay that spawned a whole discipline of the anthropology of the body. In this essay he says how he was first interested in body techniques after reading an essay in *Encyclopaedia Britannica* on swimming. He realised that there were many ways of swimming and that it had a history and indeed an anthropology. He began classifying body techniques such as how one walks, sits, rests, makes love, eats, shits etc. How and whether these are taught may have profound psycho-physical effects on behaviour. His most famous example concerns the way babies are held by their mothers, especially comparing Asian and European practices. This may in turn affect whether a person can in later life sit crossed legged or squat by a camp fire. If you doubt the usefulness of being able to squat, try a winter ritual in the woods, when the ground is too wet to sit on. Mauss studied Taoism and Hinduism and drew the tentative conclusion that body techniques may well be a necessary condition of certain mystical states.

Serpent Power

mysterious connections arise between parts of the body during sexual arousal. More than a thousand years ago, tantrik adepts described such phenomena and personified them as the goddess Kundalini. She represents the mysterious serpentine energy that lies latent in every individual. The goddess Kundalini lives in the temple called the human body. The tantriks were well aware of the physical anatomy as they were great admirers of the Ayurvedic medical system[3]. However they posited the existence of a special esoteric anatomy which supplements the more orthodox Ayurvedic conception and which was the domain of the goddess Kundalini. This tantrik esoteric anatomy has a half dozen or so key spheres of existence called chakras in Sanskrit. These are connected by three channels called nadis. Before this tantrik model became widely disseminated in the west, it was more common to use kabbalistic concepts to describe the same sort of things. Kabbalistic concepts gave magicians a unique insight into the tantrik system (and vice versa), and they were able eventually to grasp some of its significance of the tantrik magical system.[4]

One of the most useful books on this subject is still Arthur Avalon's (or Sir John Woodroffe's) *The Serpent Power - The Secrets of Tantric and Shaktic Yoga*. Most people find this a difficult book to read because of the preponderance of Sanskrit technical terms. Bharati, the highly rated scholar of tantrism, is very dismissive of Woodroffe's work although the book is often still recommended in academic circles probably because there has been very little else available.[5] I like Woodroffe because he does present some interesting primary texts without trying too hard to translate the Sanskrit technical terms in to the buzzwords of his day. The fact that many of its concepts are unique to India, makes it such a crucial area to study. Take for example a very famous term like 'atman', which is often translated by the western

---

[3] See Kris Morgan, *Medicine of the Gods* (Mandrake of Oxford 1994)
[4] The kabbalistic doctrine of seven palaces bears comparison with the chakra system and may be derived from it.
[5] A Bharati, (pseudonym of Leopold Fischer) *The Tantric Tradition*, (Rider 1970)

Sexual Magick

concept 'soul'. But this gives a misleading impression of the real meaning of âtman. This confusion arises because the line between the soul or âtman and the physical is drawn differently in the Indian tradition than it is in western theology and philosophy. The western view is derived in part from Plato and Descartes and sees the soul as a kind of ghostly intelligence. The Indian version is derived from the ancient Sankhya-yoga philosophy which makes a finer distinction between the ghostly astral body and beyond that a further transcendental essence called the âtman (or sometimes purusha).[6]

I've made this long digression in order to try to explain why Woodroffe's book has lasted the test of time. He does not try to translate unique Sanskrit terms into rough English equivalents. If he had he would undoubtedly have translated words like 'akasha' into Victorian quasi-scientific concepts like 'ether'.

Following on from this is a point often made by Mike Magee of the Kaula Nath Clan AMOOKOS. He says that these texts are only obscure because there are no gurus to explain them and teach the real practice. This begs the question that if the chakra system is so significant why have all the gurus needed to explain it disappeared from India? And why is tantra in such a decline? In trying to revive a system on the basis of translation, might we be flogging a dead horse?

On the subject of literature a few other useful books in a mass of useless ones are Crowley's *Magick*, which has a passable introduction to yoga as long as you avoid some of his more extreme notions. You could also have a look at Swami Vivekananda's *Raja Yoga* which is the source of many of Crowley's ideas on yoga.

How many chakras are there?

In the introduction to *The Serpent Power*, Arthur Avalon treats us to a humorous and scathing review of C W Leadbeater's book *The Inner Life*. Leadbeater was a well-known (perhaps even notorious)

---

[6] For more on Sankhya, see Kris Morgan, *Medicine of the Gods: gnosticism*.

Serpent Power

'Theosophical' author whose garbled account of what he called the 'force centres' and 'the serpent fire' has influenced many celebrated occultists ever since. On the basis of his own theory laden perception, Leadbeater substituted a six-petaled lotus at the spleen for the classical *svadhisthana* or sexual lotus and 'corrected' the number of petals in the head lotus, which he said is not a thousand but 960! He thus demonstrates his complete ignorance of the classical tantrik system, where 1000 is probably used as symbolic of magnitude and not as an actual number. The petals in the head lotus are similar to what thelemites refer to as the myriad stars in the body of Nuit.

Despite their shortcomings, many Theosophical ideals are preserved as if they are in some way authoritative and with depressing regularity new books purvey this distorted and non-magical view. Incidentally the spleen was a well known organ in Indian physical anatomy. The term 'spleen' comes from the Sanskrit 'pliha', in other words if the tantriks had thought there was a chakra in the spleen they would have said so, and they never did. In clinical medicine the spleen is said to be part of the lymphatic or immune system. I mention this only because it is not uncommon to compare the chakra system with the glands of the endocrine system, but even on these grounds the idea of a spleen chakra does not really work.

Some practitioners of complimentary medicine have added, with slightly more justification, the solar plexus to the Sanskrit chakra system. The solar or coliac plexus is a Latin anatomical term for complex of nerves radiating from the depression just below the breast bone. There are in fact many such plexuses recognized within the clinical model, although the solar plexus is the largest, which may be a reason to add it to the Sanskrit system. If it were counted as a chakra it falls between the navel and heart chakra. Personally I feel that the solar plexus fits best within the Ayurvedic system of regional anatomy, which includes over a hundred *marmas* or vulnerable points.

As a belated introduction, it might be useful to describe the tantrik system of psychic anatomy before passing on to a discussion of useful ways of working with it. It is not my intention to maintain that only one version of the system exists. In fact, the number of chakras does vary

Sexual Magick

from school to school, although the most common description is of six chakras or centres of psychic energy within the body.[7] Variations are mentioned in for example the *Saradatilaka* which names the following: Toes, Ankles, Knees, Thighs, Frenum of the Foreskin, Genitals, Navel, Heart, Neck, Throat, Base of the Palate, Point between the Eyebrows, Forehead, Crown and 'Brahmarandhra' (Exit to Brahman).[8] There is also a very old text within the Nath tradition which mentions eleven chakras.[9]

However the most universal system still seems to be of six chakras as found in the *Sat-Chakra-Nirupana*, which means 'investigation of the six chakras', the name of the text that is published under the title the *Serpent Power* although the translated Sanskrit text only occupies one hundred and fifty of the book's five hundred odd pages. The remainder is Woodroffe's detailed and at times dry commentary.

Most of this text concerns detailed descriptions of the chakras and very little of Kundalini herself. This is an important point and perhaps signifies that the system is to be taken as a whole and work with it includes visualization of the six chakras as much as the more glamorous 'Kundalini'. This brings to mind the doctrine of the Kabbalah where I believe the spheres are more important than the paths. The Sanskrit *Serpent Power* text concerns the eruption and experience of strange energies within the body, some in the form of chakras and some as a release of what we might call *serpentine* energy.

The Six chakras are:

Muladhara (Root). Actually this is two words - Mula[10] and Adhara. In the text it is simply called the Adhara lotus, meaning the root of the other six. If you call this the base chakra you may miss an

---

[7] Teun Goudrian and Sanjukta Gupta *Hindu Tantrism* (Leiden, Brill) page 172.
[8] See also Bhaskararaya Commentary on *Bhavana Upanisad* p 277.
[9] P C Bagchi (ed) *Kaulajnana Nirnaya* translated into English by Mike Magee (Prachya Prakashan 1987).
[10] As I say in the introduction, I intend to leave most Sanskrit spellings in their anglicised form, that is without diacritics.

Serpent Power

important point. Mula means root, as in root of a tree. This chakra is the root of the whole system. Sometimes people write of the chakra system as if its origin is at the apex and it somehow evolves down to its base or root. But the language used is not accidental. The metaphor of the root is a familiar one in the Hindu intellectual tradition. What is a root? It is an organic thing, something that bursts out from a seed. Kundalini is a seed within the earth. She lies dormant in the earth chakra until something or someone summons her forth. She may have been planted there by Shiva and perhaps it is he who subsequently calls her forth, bidding her form again the divine tree that leads back through its branches to him and beyond.

Svadhisthana (Sexual). This is again two words, Sva meaning own and adhisthana meaning basis. This term is applied to the creative principle with yourself (sex) and the universe (supreme or para lingam). Jung, in an interesting discussion of the tantrik chakra system,[11] says that this chakra represents the ocean of the unconscious. The sacred animal of this chakra is the Leviathan (makara[12]), the mysterious monster of the deep. This chakra is, according to Jung, thoroughly feminine and contains the mystery of the first initiation into the watery abyss.

Manipura (Navel). The navel chakra alternatively called the nabhi-chakra was described in the ancient *Yoga Sutras*.[13] It includes the stomach but also the scar left after our stay in our mother's womb and the point of contact between us. It can be concluded that the navel itself is no dead piece of flesh but retains some sympathetic links with our origins.

---

[11] In 1932 Jung gave some superior lectures entitled 'Psychological Commentary on Kundalini Yoga' which are republished in *Spring* 1975 & 1976.

[12] There is a weak pun possible here between makara and makârâ meaning the five 'm's or powerful enjoyments.

[13] Translated into Arabic in the tenth century by Albiruni and therefore maybe the source of early knowledge of the chakras.

Sexual Magick

Anahata (Heart). Hata sounds like heart but in fact the word means the region of unstruck sound. The heart is said to be the place where one can hear the unstruck or cosmic sound.[14]

Vishuddha (Throat) means literally place without impurities.

Ajna ('Third Eye'). This is the place of unlimited power and authority. Shiva lives here in his form as lord of yoga and also eroticism, he is therefore shown with an erection.

Beyond the chakras is the **Sahasrara**, which exists in the empty place (shunyadesha) above. It is common to consider this as another chakra, sometimes located at the crown of the head or perhaps more accurately as a nimbus beyond the head.

'This lotus, lustrous and whiter than the full-moon, has its head turned downwards. It charms. Its clustered filaments are tinged with the colour of the young sun. Its body is luminous with letters.'[15]

Contained within this system of six major chakras and the place beyond, is a very powerful sexual and emotional metaphor that suggests a process by which the goddess Kundalini is persuaded to climb upwards to join with Shiva in his mountain refuge. (It may also be valid to persuade Shiva to come down off his mountain and to unite with Kundalini in her forest retreat. I do not see why Sahasrara has to be fixed to any one part of space; it is up, down and enveloping the body). When Shiva and Kundalini are united, they move off together into the realm beyond the ajna chakra. Whether the practitioner of this magick is male, female or mixed, they would, in my opinion, assume the godform of Kundalini.

---

[14] Called *shabda-brahman*, a complex doctrine worthy of meditation. The old Zen koan about what is the sound of one hand clapping is answered by it.

[15] *Sat Chakra Nirupana* Vs 40

Serpent Power

Some Correspondences of the Six Chakras

Sanskrit name	English name	Element	Colour	Sacred[16] Animal
Muladhara	Root	Earth	Yellow	Elephant
Svadhisthana	Genitals	Water	Grey	Leviathan
Manipura	Navel	Fire	Red	Goat
Anahata	Chest	Air	Light Blue	Gazelle
Vishuddha	Throat	Space	Dark Blue	Elephant
Ajna	Forehead			

Thelemic magicians often compare the chakra system with the Hermetic tradition and also with the Kabbalistic Tree of Life glyph.[17] Allowing for a possible change of gender, some have seen in the verse

---

[16] Jung *op. cit.*
In the second of these he has some interesting insights to the symbolism of the sacred animals. The elephant is the most powerful of the beasts of Earth. Similarly with the Whale or *Makara* in Sanskrit. The goat is the totemic and also sacrificial animal of Agni the fire god situated in the stomach. The gazelle a suitably refined animal for the first of the subtle elements, air, which is invisible. The reappearance of the elephant is a problem for the symbolism but Jung surmises that it is the elephant in its higher spiritual guise.

[17] My own correspondence, for what its worth places Malkuth at Muladhara; Yesod at Svadhisthana; Tiphereth includes two chakras viz: Manipura and Anahata; Daath includes also two chakras viz: Vishuddha and Ajna. Sahasrara, which is, strickly speaking, not a chakra, can be compared with the supernal Kether.

Sexual Magick

quoted above a description of Nuit, the great stellar goddess who appears only when the third or magical eye is open.[18]

The Nath sect further simplifies the chakra system into three key points within the body that may be brought into balance. These three are the head, the heart and the sexual organs. Following on from the above description, it is clear that the muladhara is not the same thing as the sexual centre although it is closely associated with it. In the source text the muladhara is said to be a red flower with four petals. The red is like that of the rising sun and it is situated in the middle between the anus and the penis. These classical accounts usually describe things from a male standpoint. The practice was developed for a male worshipper and a female shakti or instrument. This is one aspect of traditional tantrism that needs re-evaluation. Inside the muladhara lotus is a yellow square, the symbol of earth which is the dominant element here. Also described are various presiding deities. One of the most important of these is Ganesha who is the gateway guardian of earth. Ganesha, the elephant-headed god, is an Indian equivalent of Hermes. Both gods are associated with serpentine energy - Ganesha's trunk is like a snake and he wears a 'sacred thread' but unlike the brahmanical variety, his is made of a living snake. Hermes too has a wand or caduceus constructed of living serpents. Hermes and Ganesha are both threshold guardians and should always be worshipped before any other act of Magick.

If Ganesha lets you into the earth chakra, in some sense one is also at a specific sacred site or its equivalent within the body, a topic to be discussed in the next chapter. This place is called *Kamarupa*, 'the place of desire', whose outer manifestation is to be found in Assam in modern India.

At *Kamarupa* is a phallic symbol of Shiva, not crafted by any human hand, but one that has generated itself. Covering this phallic stone or situated nearby is the object of many magician's quest - the mystic Kundalini. She is said to be

---

[18] Undoubtedly there is a sexual mystery here, as Jung thought that a single eye was a metaphor for human sexuality.

Serpent Power

'fine as a fibre of lotus stalk, She is the Goddess Maya (of uncanny power), who bewilders the created. She covers the mouth of the phallic stone with her own mouth and is coiled around it three and a half times, like a sleeping snake. Her murmur sounds like the drone of innumerable intoxicated bees.'[19]

This is an extremely rich and evocative symbol. The ancient Hindus were well aware of its multilayered nature. Not every detail is to be taken literally and you shouldn't expect there to be an actual serpent. There is a fascinating book on this subject of serpents, called *Indian Serpent Lore - or The Nagas in Hindu Legend and Art*.[20] India is fortunate in having one of the best documented traditions of serpent worship, continuing up to the present day amongst the rural population of the Punjab Hills. These divine serpents or Nagas share some characteristics with werewolves in that they can change shape into human form at will. In the legends they only assume their true serpentine form when either asleep or having sexual intercourse! Snakes are often associated with the earth, where they are found guarding 'phallic' ant-hills full of treasure. The legend of the Nagas is like the medieval European legend of the water sprite Melusina, who turned into a serpent once a year.[21]

The English word 'serpent' may well derive from the Sanskrit 'sarpa', which describes its peculiar writhing movements. The snake is a potent symbol of a special type of energy found within the earth and in our own bodies. If the sleeping Kundalini is aroused, she will discard her serpentine form and take on that of a Goddess. Thus she is described differently in each of the chakras or places she passes through. Parallel to this are the transformations of Shiva. When Shiva sleeps he sometimes takes on the form of a phallic stone.

---

19 Avalon, *op cit.*
20 J Ph Vogel *Indian Serpent Lore* (Probsthain 1926). Also E C Dimock 'Goddess of Snakes in Medeival Bengali Literature' *Journal History of Religions*, (University of Chicago 1964).
21 Sabine Baring-Gould *Curious Myths of the Middle Ages* (Jupiter Books 1977).

Some people say that Crowley was describing Kundalini in the follwing passage from *Liber Al*:

'I am the secret Serpent coiled about to spring: in my coiling there is joy. If I lift up my head, I and my Nuit are one. If I droop down my head, and shoot forth venom, then is the rapture of the earth, and I and the earth are one.' Al II.26.

If this is Kundalini then the gender has been changed, Crowley's serpent power is male. A technique for working with this energy is described in one of the appendices to *Magick*[22] although a great deal of the symbolism employed by Crowley is very personal to him.

Common Experience of the Chakras

Even before you start practising tantrik body magick, you will have had some experience of the chakras, because they are, in my opinion, manifested in some very familiar bodily sensations. The chakras have something in them of some very familiar bodily sensations, all connected with the emotions. The Muladhara or root chakra corresponds to a visceral sensation of fear. Experience shows that fear is a potent way of arousing the body's energy.

The Svadhisthana or sexual centre is connected with sexual feelings.

The Manipura or stomach is connected with nervousness and fear.

The Anahata or heart chakra is connected with strong emotions, especially love.

The Vishuddha or throat centre with emotional upset.

These everyday experiences give a clue to the existence of an entire system within the body linked to the emotions. The simple observation of these facts are what probably lead on to the more elaborate system of esoteric tantrism.

We are of course all looking for a more intense and transforming experience of our body's psychic centres. For this you need various other techniques or practices such as those mentioned in the magical

---

[22] Appendix VII, *Liber HHH*, page 362 in 1929 edition.

and yogic literature. They fall into two groups: the yogic and the symbolic.

Yogic Techniques

Under Yoga can be included any physical activity or technique that either deliberately or spontaneously causes these strange bodily sensations to occur. Strictly Yogic techniques usually involve control of the vital airs (prana) and an elaborate physiological explanation of what is happening. The world's most famous Yogi is for many B. K. S. Iyengar whose *Light On Yoga* is a modern classic. In the introduction to the lotus pose he translates a section from the *Hatha Yoga Pradipika*:

'Assuming the lotus pose and having placed the palms one upon the other, fix the chin firmly upon the breast and contemplating upon Brahman, frequently contract the anus and raise the apana or down breath up; by similar contraction of the throat force the prana (up breath) down. By this he obtains unequalled knowledge through the favour of Kundalini (which is roused by this process.'[23]

Many magicians have tried something like this and here is an extract from my own magical diary:

'I experienced something like [the above] very soon after I had first began the serious study of Magick. I was working my way through Crowley's *Magick In Theory & Practice* and Vivekananda's *Raja Yoga*. I spent about a month trying to master my posture which had been very bad.[24] One night I sat in my temple breathing slowly and concentrating hard. I felt a rush of energy in my heart and throat, an experience so difficult to describe that I can understand why people use so many symbols. It was an ecstatic bursting forth of joy, with a focus in my throat,

---

23 B K S Iyengar *Light On Yoga* (Allen & Unwin 1968) Page 97.
24 On the subject of posture I would recommend Padmasana (cross-legged) rather than Virasana (kneeling), as it brings the Muladhara Chakra into a closer contact with the ground.

Sexual Magick

which felt like it had never felt before. After a few minutes I had to stop the exercise as I thought it was going to kill me. However I now regret stopping and wish I had trusted my body and followed it through - easier said than done.'

Symbolic Arousal

This involves a mixture of the sort of physical techniques mentioned above, with the addition of symbolism and ritual. Kenneth Grant claims that there is a difference in quality between Kundalini aroused in the symbolic way and that done using the Yogic techniques. He believes that *imaginatively* aroused Kundalini is somehow 'safer' than that which is aroused *physically*. Personally I doubt if this distinction is genuine; in fact such a division between the psychic and the somatic is alien to Indian thought.[25] The tantriks recommend a mixture of visualization, breathing and posture as the more potent technique and often disparage the purely physical approach.

Arousal of Kundalini by symbolic methods occurs during a well conducted ritual, especially during the invocation, which can literally make the hair stand on end. Some people may even have experienced this during Christian rituals. Sanskrit poetics is especially concerned with creating a pattern of words that is able to evoke spiritual changes in the hearer. The ability of a poem to create this kind of response is a question of taste.[26] A text that I found very profound comes from the *Brihadaranyaka Upanishad* VI.i and concerns prana or the bodily airs:

7. These bodily organs (prana) were disputing among themselves, each vaunting its own superiority. They went to Brahman and asked him which of them was the best. He replied: 'That one is the best on whose departure the body seems to be at its worst.'

---

[25] Kris Morgan 'Catharsis' *Celtic Dawn II* Sept 1988.
[26] Taste or *rasa* in the tantrik/ayurvedic tradition is a subject worthy of study by the magician. For a start, see Kris Morgan, *Medicine of the Gods*.

Serpent Power
8. The voice went off and stayed away for a year. On its return it said: 'How did you manage without me?' They replied 'We were like the dumb, not speaking with the voice, but breathing with the breath, seeing with the eye, hearing with the ear, knowing with the mind, begetting with the semen. That is how we lived.' The voice entered the body again........
So each in turn left the body for a year until it came to breath's turn.
13. The breath of life was on the point of going off. As a great and goodly stallion from the Indus country might tear up the pegs to which it is tethered all together, so was the breath of life (on the point of) tearing up the (other) bodily organs. They said: 'Good sir, do not go away; for we will never manage to live without you.' 'Then make me an offering,' said the breath of life. 'So be it.' (said they).

Symbolic arousal of Kundalini might be achieved by an extension of the astral temple meditation mentioned briefly earlier. This may be familiar to experienced magicians as the Malkuth temple meditation. This version is based upon the Shri yantra diagram and the Body Yantra meditation given in AMOOKOS's *Tantra Magick*. If you are quite familiar with this kind of exercise then you can safely skip the next few pages: the extension I suggest comes after the operator has mastered, usually over the course of a year's magical work, the elemental parts of the *temple of desire* or Kamarupa. He or she will have noticed that the first shrine room contains a sealed room whose entrance is immediately behind the central Shiva lingam. You may already have guessed that the Goddess Kundalini lies immediately behind these doors and may at the appropriate time be invoked here. For some this happens spontaneously, but in the main I recommend that you do not pass onto this part of the ritual until you have really mastered the elemental work. But the choice is yours, the risk is either too rapid an advancement or worse still, that you have insufficient momentum to make the meditation work and it becomes a damp squib.

The Kamarupa Temple Meditation

Preamble

Here is a concept in Magick whose importance cannot be overemphasised - the construction of a imaginary counterpart to your physical temple.[27]

Every style of Magick has its own particular astral temple. In Kabbalah I have heard it called the Malkuth temple, and its description is based upon the mystical drawing called the Tree of Life. In Chaos Magick it is the Chaos Sphere; in Greek Magick is the Tetratis. In Thelema the astal temple could well be based on the description given in *Liber Al* I.51.[28] The Renaissance magus Giordano Bruno coined the term 'Theatre of Memory' for this concept. He designed, in his mind's eye, an imaginary Greek theatre, where every part had symbolic significance. He could use this technique to memorise the relationship between very complex groups of symbols. Similar images were used by John Dee and Robert Fludd, see for instance Palladio's reconstruction

---

[27] The Islamic scholar Henry Corbin has written a very interesting essay on the power of the myth of the lost or destroyed temple. He begins with a quote from the Talmud, which says that when the Romans destroyed the second temple, it was a disaster not merely for the Jews but for the whole human race. Actually the real disaster may have occurred when Nebuchadnezzar burnt the first Solomonic temple and the priests returned the keys to the angelic beings, thus breaking one of the last direct links between Gods and humanity. This is a recurrent myth, one in which the earth no longer contains the divine temple but has become its crypt. This myth contains within it the entire aim of magick. See Henry Corbin, 'L'Imago Templi', *Spring* Vol 43 (1974); 'La Configuration du Temple de la Ka'ba comme secret de la vie spirituelle' Spring, Vol 34 (1965). Both these articles are in English and ar reprinted in his *Eranos-Jahrbuch*.

[28] This insight comes from Stephen Ashe 'Liber Al and the Fifty Gates of Babalon' reprinted in *Thelema XC (1994) - Proceedings of the Ninth International Symposium of Thelemic Magick*.

Serpent Power

of the theatre of Vitruvious or even the plans of Shakespeare's Globe theatre.[29] This is a very important discovery.

The basic design of the tantrik astral temple is the Shri Yantra, the most famous and universal of all the mystical diagrams (mandala or yantra). If you are not familiar with this diagram, then it is reproduced on page 85 of *Tantra Magick* in bare outline, and elsewhere throughout that book in various sections and partial views. I am indebted to blessed Ganesha, the Elephant headed one, for revealing to me some of its significance.

Becoming familiar with the lineaments of the astral temple, is usually accomplished by the repeated practice of guided visualisation or so-called 'pathworking'. This is where the experimenter imagines him or herself walking or moving through the designated landscape or building in serial order. Thus at first only the lower parts of the glyph are traversed, building up a great familiarity with its topography. As one grows in mental stamina and ability, higher and higher levels of the glyph are opened up to the explorer.

It is possible to obtain pre-recorded tapes of famous pathworkings, which are designed so that the experimenter may follow the imagery as it unfolds. In my experience this kind of pre-recorded guided visualisation is of limited use. The more the experimenter gets into the pathworking, the more distracting becomes the voice on the tape. The speaker may insist that the statue has an angry face, when you've already seen it, and it is smiling! The answer is perhaps to read (or play) the description once or twice, and then do the pathworking without the tape. Alternatively the guide can lead you to a particular door, describing what is behind the door and then invite you to step through it alone, and explore it at your own pace. The guide then remains silent - the best examples of this are done in rituals, and the guide has been chosen beforehand and will often not read from a prearranged script but will improvise with what comes into their head, a kind of stream of consciousness. When the guide stops talking, the group can lapse into their own meditation or pathworking. So what the

---

[29] See Francis Yates, *The Art of Memory*.

Sexual Magick

guide is saying is not scripted, it is what they are 'seeing' or intuiting - they are in fact in a low level trance, which can often deepen significantly when they lapse into silence.

When the guide invites you to proceed on your own, do so. Follow the vision, however feeble, to its natural conclusion. The session usually terminates when you reach your goal or begin to run out of mental stamina and feel the need to wind things up. During this time, you may have become quite dissociated from your physical body. Perhaps it is some physical sensation, such as pins and needles that disturbs you, or the subtle movements of others in the room who have obviously finished. Alternatively, you may hear a gentle sounding of a bell chimed by one of the other participants, as the pre-arranged signal to return. When either of these things happens, try and mentally retrace your steps to where the guided visualisation began. When you have done this, become fully aware of your body again and if necessary vibrate or chant some sacred words to really ground yourself. It is especially important to join in with any chanting at the end of the ritual where appropriate, or do your closing, as this serves to balance everything up again and prevent unwanted obsession.

Transition

You need to develop an image that represents the transition from your normal mindscape to that of the astral temple. To do this you must accept the following fantasy - your temple room or bedroom is an individual 'cell' in a vast oriental monastery (vihara). When you have done your opening rite, settle down and close your eyes. 'Look' around your room in your mind's eye and see the changes. The honey coloured stone walls of a building, which you know you have never been in before and yet seems familiar. You see the door by which you came in, but also a curtain hand-woven from three fabrics, one is browny red, the other is white and the third is black. Imagine yourself approaching this curtain, but before touching it, trace the symbol of earth[30] upon it and then draw it aside. Behind this is an old wooden door, with a bolt

---

[30] Choose this for yourself, I use an equal armed cross in a circle.

Serpent Power

and padlock. You remember that you have a key to the padlock around your neck. Unlock and open the door.

Look around.

You are in a very large enclosure in blazing sunlight. It is the courtyard of a Hindu temple. You may be able to see its honey coloured outer walls of stone. They are at least twenty feet high and should remind you of a Moorish castle, with crenelations.

How large is the space? I think it is very large, I designed it so. The total space enclosed by these walls is about that of a football pitch. Beyond them you can see a very high range of mountains, which surrounds on all sides the valley in which this temple is built. Beyond the mountains you see sky and clouds. This is an incredibly safe place for you. Nothing in this enclosure can ever harm you. Whenever you have need of sanctuary on an inner level, this is the image to call to mind. Take some time to wander around the enclosure, taking note of some of these details, and recording them in your magical diary. The following details are especially interesting (to me at least):

What time of day is it?
What season of the year it?
What kind of weather can you see?
Are there any other people you can see?
Do any supernatural beings appear, if so what happens?
When you first 'see' the courtyard of your astral temple, where are you, i.e. east, west, north south, whatever?

[By the way, if you feel you've 'seen' enough and really need to stop, simply go back to the door and curtain (your deep mind will know where it is) visualise it one last time, pass through it back into your meditation room. Sit down. Visualise the seal of earth glowing on the curtain cloth then fading and come back to yourself, as before. Vibrate OM three times to really ground yourself.]

If you are ready to see the rest of the temple, this is some of what can been seen:

You are standing in the east, facing west. Before you rises the massive central tower of the temple of Kamarupa. It is fantastic and you must crane your neck to see the top, where the rays of sunlight

Sexual Magick

bounce off golden stonework. This temple complex is brand new - you can tell this because many of the places for carvings have been left blank, awaiting completion. The tower is covered with many unfinished carvings or blank spaces ready for carving. There will be so many images of gods and goddess when the temple is finished, you wonder how you will ever make sense of it.

You look before you at ground level and see, set to one side, a square communal bathing place, with seven steps leading down to the murky water. But before you can go there, you must pay the bath keeper.

Look at the Bath keeper.

With a nod of recognition you see the elephant headed god, Ganesha. You push a coin into his hand, and he invites you to continue. You walk slowly down the seven steps, removing your clothing as you go. In the water you can see frogs and other creatures, probably fish, swimming there. You see a shoal of fish moving together, then breaking the surface of the water with their heads, looking for a moment, then dashing off under the surface. You wash away your memories in the water of forgetfulness, wash away the worry and problems of the mundane world. When you finish, you step out of the waist-deep water on the other side, someone hands you some clean clothes. Now you can walk up the steps and into the eastern doorway of the tower. You climb up twenty-five steps until you can enter the first shrine room. This room is a massive but regular cube, perhaps 30 feet by 30 feet by 30 feet. In the centre is a low, stone altar, perfectly square on two of its sides, but about two feet high. In the centre is a giant stone lingam, resting in a yoni. The stone is black, granite like, polished by the hands of many millions of pilgrims. You see the offerings of those past pilgrims - tiny flower petals. You have a moment alone, and can leave an offering if you have one, perhaps offering the things you have achieved today. This offering could also be in the form of a flower petal. Before leaving it you must breathe

Serpent Power

some of your spirit into it using the tantrik nyasa technique[31] and then place it gently on the lingam. Before passing on, you take the hem of your garment and polish the black stone. When you do this, observe how that object changes or reacts, if at all.

Your devotion finished, you circumambulate the shrine. In the South and Northern sides, a window has been cut, and you can see out across the enclosure, across the temple's outer walls, to the landscape beyond. Through the southern window you see many things, but mainly the line of high mountains, the highest in the world. And amongst them in the south you see the smoking peak of an active volcano.

In the west is another doorway, its way guarded by priests who smile at someone who is standing just behind you, but will not let you past. You see beyond them another room, dark and lit by lamps and full of strange unfamiliar things. Some light comes in through another window, opening to the west and you can perhaps see through it to the mountains beyond and just glimpse the reflection of a distant lake beneath the far mountains. You pass on around the shrine reaching the north, you again look out and see only mountains, dark and brooding. You guess that here there would be a deep cave, leading to the bowels of the earth. As you pass back to the eastern doorway, a priest smiles at you and offers you a small round ball of some eatable, you fold this carefully in your clothes and pass on. Pause on the top of the stairway, you see again the bath below you, and beyond that the mountains to the east, the highest of all, and one in particular, towering above anything you have ever seen. It breaks through the clouds, and strong winds rush over it. Take a few moments to absorb the sight and then climb down.

Now if you wish, you may return again to whence you came back to your meditation room and waiting body. Every day of your practice

---

[31] Nyasa - placing. In simplest form, visualise your self-chosen deity appearing in the region of your heart. When this is clear, imagine that it begins to move in time with your in and out breath. With each breath it moves a little further, until you breathe it out through your left nostril and 'catch' it on a prepared flower petal and can then gently guide it to the image. At the end of the ritual, reverse this process.

Sexual Magick

you should aim to return to the temple, make your oblation to the stone lingam and yoni, receive your gift from the temple (prasad) and return. Each time note whether anything has changed. Does anyone say anything to you, do any strange things happen? Note it all down in your diary, how do you feel?

Do not expect the image to be very sharp at this stage. Your powers of visualisation may be very feeble, but they will develop if you give them a chance. Even if it seems that you are 'making' it happen, and that most of your mind is still very much rooted in the real world, try to go with it, like a favourite daydream.

The Kalas

In the 1970, Kenneth Grant wrote a book about Crowley that did much to awaken interest in the tantrik current within Thelemic magick. The book was called *Aleister Crowley and the Hidden God* and it contains an account of the system called the kalas, thought by many to be an extension of the tantrik Kundalini yoga. Kala means part or aspect, and is used in tantrik literature to refer to the subsidiary aspects of the primal goddess, for example those corresponding to the eight petals on the Shri Yantra, or in an example given by Bharati, ten aspects arranged on the intersecting triangles of the yantra.[32] Another important meaning of kala is in Kalyanamalla's *Anangaranga* or *Arena of the Love God*. This book was written in the sixteenth century as a updated version of the *Kamasutra*, written sometime between the second century BCE and the second century CE. Whilst the *Kamasutra* contains many important sexual magick themes, including body piercing and body striking, it is on the whole a manual of courtly love. It was clearly written before tantrism was created or rediscovered (whichever theory you prefer). The *Anangaranga*, on the other hand was written after tantrism had reached its zenith and therefore contains many tantrik ideas. Like many ancient erotic texts they are written by men observing women and they can seem cold and clinical. It is hard to imagine real sexual beings consulting the calendar before they make

---

[32] Bharati (1970) p. 254 and footnote 59.

love in order to work out which part of their lover's body they should caress. These reservations aside, we can say that the core of erotic texts like the *Anangaranga* stem from the observations all lovers naturally make of the ebb and flow of desire and the variations through the day, month and year in the way one experiences a lover's body. This may include changes in taste, feel, smell etc. Anyway, for what its worth here is the section in the *Anangaranga* that details some of these variations. I would suggest that a matrix could also be drawn up for a man's body, I would welcome the reader's own observations on this.

1. Speaking generally from the full moon day the Chandrakala[33] descends by the left side of the woman from the forehead through the eyes, cheeks, lips, chin, neck, shoulder, arm-pit, breast, the side, hip, public region, genitals, knee, ankle and foot; on the new moon day it starts the upward course by the right side in a like manner and reaches the forehead on the full moon day.

2-3. When the position of the Chandrakala in a woman is in her scalp, her passion should be roused by gently touching the hair like a comb; if it is in the eyes, cheeks and lips then these should be kissed passionately; if it is in her neck or arm-pit, it should be marked with your fingernail. If in the breast, waist, side and hip these should be pressed with firm hands. The navel should be petted with your palm, if in the genitals the tongue should be pressed inside the vagina and it should be sucked. If in the chest it should be gently struck, public region with your own pubis, thumb with your thumb, feet should be pressed with your feet. By arousing the erogenous zones a man who is well versed in the art of love will capture a woman's heart and both will derive maximum pleasure.'

---

[33] Means literally moon-period or time although usually translated as erogenous zone. The allusion is to the daily waxing or waning of the moon. Sexual desire is likened to a moon, centred in the head, that over the course of a month waxes bigger, moving down through the body until it reaches its peak at the vagina. As the moon wanes, so too does the Kala, retreating upward through the body.

Sexual Magick

There then follows a passage that details some variations to this basic pattern, supposedly determined by the psychological and physical characteristics of women. The author gives a fourfold classification, supposedly in descending order from the Lotus woman, Picture woman, Conch woman and Elephant woman. There is no equivalent classification given to men. This is a clue that the above section is an interpolation perhaps from another text. In the next chapter the author provides a totally different trifold classification of men and women, which is similar to the Ayurvedic trifold classifying of bodily types.[34] The *Anangaranga* here classifies men and women according to genital size. Men are said to be either Rabbit, Bull or Horse type, approximately twelve, eighteen or twenty four centimetres respectively. For women the types are Deer, Mare and Elephant and the internal dimensions are said to be the same. Equal unions e.g. between Rabbit and Deer are said to be excellent. Controversially the text then goes on to classify a *higher* form of sexual union obtainable *only* when a horse man and a deer woman unite.

You might think this is a slightly offensive but purely historical relic of sexuality, but it is surprising how these things cling on. Witness for example the number of jokes in popular films and television about genital size, usually aimed at men. Men find this a difficult issue to deal with, as I suppose women would if the corresponding doctrine on vaginal size received similar attention. There are large, so called 'elephant' women who do not have corresponding massive vaginas, likewise there are large men who have small penises. It's worth repeating that the kind of mechanistic approach to lovemaking that is captured in the ancient Indian erotic text has no real part in the modern world.

---

[34] See Kris Morgan, *Medicine of the Gods* (Mandrake 1994) p. 31ff.

Kundalini and Wilheim Reich

At the risk of seeming a bit hackneyed I'd like to finish this chapter with a brief mention of Wilhelm Reich.[35] One of the most important books of the twentieth century must surely be Reich's *The Function of the Orgasm*. Mike Magee has done a great deal to rekindle interest in Reich by drawing attention to the parallels between his views and those of tantrik magick. Reich was on his own admission hostile to 'yoga' and things Indian; despite this his discovery of a blue bio-energy is very suggestive of Kundalini herself. Rather than try to summarize Reich it is best to read it for oneself; here is a remarkable passage from one of his case notes:

> 'Following the consistent description of the rigid attitude of his mouth, a clonic twitching of his lips set in, weak at first but growing gradually stronger. He was surprised by the involuntary nature of this twitching and defended himself against it. I told him to give into every impulse. Thereupon, his lips began to protrude and retract rhythmically and to hold the protruded position for several seconds as if in a tonic spasm. In the course of these movements, his face took on the unmistakable expression of an infant. The patient was startled, grew fearful, and asked me what this might lead to. I allayed his fears and asked him to continue to give in to every impulse and to tell me whenever he sensed the inhibition of an impulse.'

The therapy continued over several sessions:

> 'Roughly four weeks elapsed before the following took place: the twitching of various parts of his body lost more and more their spasmodic tonic character. The clonus also diminished and strange twitching appeared in the abdomen. They were not new to me, for I had seen them in many other patients, but not in connection in which they now revealed themselves. The upper part of his body jerked forward, the middle of his abdomen remained still, and the

---

[35] A superior article on Reich is to be found in *Nuit Isis* Volume one entitled '*WR - Tantrik Saint.*'

Sexual Magick

lower part of his body jerked toward the upper part. The entire response was an organic unitary movement. There were sessions in which this movement was repeated continuously. Alternating with this jerking of his entire body, there were sensations of *current* in some parts of his body, particularly in his legs and abdomen, which he experienced as pleasurable. The attitude of his mouth and face changed a little. In one such attack, his face had the unmistakable expression of a fish. Without any prompting on my part, before I had drawn his attention to it, the patient said, "I feel like a primordial animal," and shortly afterwards "I feel like a fish." [36]

These passages won't tally with everyone's experience for obvious reasons; each individual 'character armour' is different. The sort of experience described seems to belong to the crude beginnings of tantrik yoga, where the body's latent vibrancy is first aroused. When the first shock passes and the paths of inner energy smoothed, (in Yogic terms, the channels purified by breath control) one reaches a plateau of alert receptiveness. This is what Reichians call vibrancy. The magician goes on from here to work on the movements of the current of energy mentioned in the Reichian passages, which were described almost 1500 years earlier in tantrik sources.

There are several good manuals around that contain simple exercises for sensing of one's bio-energy. Many of them appear to be adaptations of Yogic *bandhas* or locks. In order to try this one should stand comfortably with the feet parallel with the body. Hold the hands, palms together opposite the chest. Press the finger tips firmly together and if you are supple enough rotate your hands so that the finger-tips are facing the chest. Keep this rather awkward position for a few minutes, breathing naturally. When you have had enough, bring the finger tips back to their original position and slowly release the pressure. Gently move the palms of your hands apart until there is a space of about one inch between them. You should sense a flow of

---

[36] Wilhelm Reich *The Function of the Orgasm* Pages 311 & 321 (English translation).

Serpent Power

energy between your two hands. For further exercises see Alexander Lowen and Leslie Lowen's *The Way to Vibrant Health*. [37]

Before I began the study of magick I was a very armoured individual. I had many personal taboos and inhibitions about my sexuality. I have made some progress but am not yet where I think I need to be. It was in fact problems with my own sexual identity that led me into the study of magick in the first place. Finding the works of Aleister Crowley at an early point in my journey of discovery was a baptism by fire. From Crowley I learnt to stop wanting to be normal and to see that part of me which is most unique as also me at my most human. I hope you will go the same way.

---

[37] Alexander Lowen and Leslie Lowen's *The Way to Vibrant Health* (Harper & Row 1977).

3
As Brothers Fight Ye![1]

Mysteries of Seth

The sixth trump in the Crowley-Harris Tarot deck or *Book of Thoth* is the Lovers or Brothers: a card which Crowley says in the text to accompany the *Book of Thoth*, is one of the most obscure and difficult of the whole pack. This card has particular significance to Thelemites and it has been claimed that the twins are the two aspects of Horus alluded to in *Liber Al*. It is my contention that one possible insight into the meaning of this card is to see it as the Lovers *and* the Brothers. The two brothers in question are Seth and Horus, who are actually represented in the card by the figures of Cain and Abel, sons of Lilith and Eve respectively. The sexual conflict between Seth and Horus and its implications for magick is to be discussed below.

It is well known that Aleister Crowley the inspiration for a great number of modern occultists, developed a whole magical theory and practice out of his own bisexuality. This kind of Magick is usually

---

[1] The title of this chapter is a quote from *Liber AL* III, 59. An earlier version of the talk was published in *NUIT ISIS* #4 Spring Equinox 1988

associated with the formula of the number eleven. Eleven is of course a number with particular significance to all Thelemites, one could almost say that the symbolism of the number eleven lies at the heart of all Thelemic Magick, indeed that eleven is the number of Magick or as it says in *Liber Al* 'My number is 11, as all their numbers who are of us.'[2]. It is possible to analyse the meaning of the number eleven on many different levels, numerical and symbolic. For instance meditate upon the shape of two upright strokes on the page - one plus one. Compare this with one plus zero. As symbols the two strokes could represent two erect phalli or two vulvas side by side; just as one and zero could represent a phallus and a vulva side by side. This is a valid way of inferring something of the magical meaning of any number. On this intuitive level eleven must have some connection with the homo-erotic kind of magick.

Kenneth Grant is a very interesting writer but he has in my opinion attempted to avoid the implications of the number eleven in magick. In Kenneth Grant's *Aleister Crowley and the Hidden God* he says that

> 'The ancient Draconian mysteries . . . are silent concerning any sodomitical formula except as a perversion of Magical practice.'[3].

Are we then to believe that Crowley somehow made a big mistake when he taught that modern magick must include, as indeed it has always included, a homosexual mystery? I think not. Uncomfortable as it may be, it is my contention that Crowley was on very strong ground when he recognised the importance of the homo-erotic current.[4] His own bisexuality made him more open to the possibilities, but he was also keying in to a very ancient tradition within magick itself. Indeed it may well have been that in the past, homosexuality was a sufficiently

---

2   *Liber Al* I, 60
3   Kenneth Grant *Aleister Crowley and the Hidden God* (Muller 1973) Page 109.
4   See Randy Conner, *Blossom of Bone - Reclaiming the connection between Homo-eroticism and the sacred.* (Harper Collins 1993).

As Brothers Fight Ye!

strange and ambiguous psychological state so as to act as a mark[5] that someone truly was a magician. Nowadays we need not go that far, but we can say that being a homosexual certainly doesn't bar a person from magick and indeed it has its own mystery. Some magicians may be temperamentally unable to explore this path for themselves but that is no reason to disapprove of others so doing. It could also be that all magicians, whatever their temperament, should at least be able to contemplate, even as a thought experiment, the possibility of a homosexual act. Not to be able to even think about it, shows in my opinion a block that needs removing.

In one of the appendices of Crowley's *Magick* is a document called *Liber O*. This contains a number of elementary Magical exercises, and the text is derived from material taught to members of the Hermetic Order of the Golden Dawn. One of the most important of these exercises is the assumption of God forms. In this key exercise the student is recommended to study the characteristic postures of the Gods, especially those of ancient Egypt; these postures should then be duplicated by the Magician. There is a crucial Magical point made by this practice - that by emulating the master one becomes the master. For example when in the banishing ritual of the pentagram you adopt the characteristic posture of Osiris, as seen in countless images of this God, so that thereby you channel some of his power and majesty into the ritual. In this way those pictures of the Gods that have come down to us from antiquity are said to be visible representations of a physical technique. By mediating upon and studying these pictures the magicians can intuitively reconstruct one of the lost techniques of Magick.[6] Pictures of the gods are one of the methods by which magical techniques are communicated.[7]

---

5   In the past magicians were expected to exhibit physical marks of their specialness. e.g. the Buddha had birthmarks on the soles of his feet.
6   A similar thing is possible for those images from non-literate cultures of our past such as the Palaeolithic, whose gods have been called the forgotten ones.
7   A Bharati, in his book *The Tantric Tradition*, makes similar deductions from Hindu and Buddhist religious art. The Yab-Yum posture of

As Brothers Fight Ye!

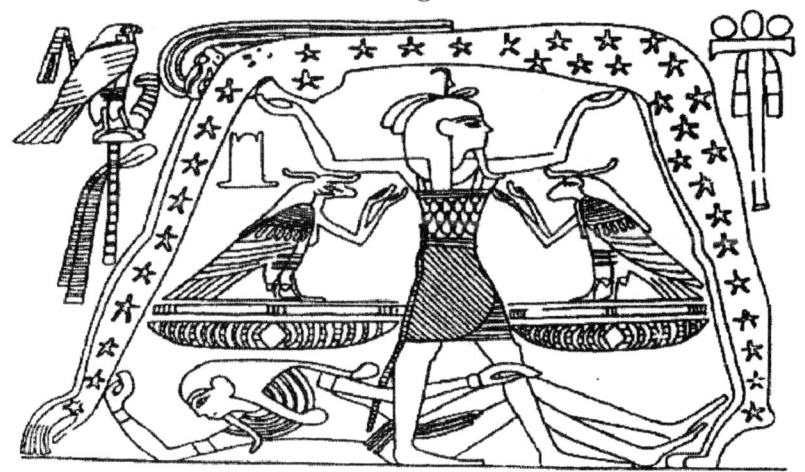

Nuit: 'her mouth is the western horizon, her vulva is the eastern horizon' from a coffin in the Rijks-Museum, Leiden

Much has been made in Thelemic circles, of the pictorial glyph of the *Stele of Revealing*. This shows the priest Ankh-f-n-Khonsu, making an offering to Horus. Arching above them is the goddess Nuit, and flying up towards her navel or womb is the winged sun. Nuit is adopting a certain posture and in other similar pictures, the winged sun is replaced by the earth god Geb, and instead of a winged sun, he is shown with his erect phallus reaching up for union, or indeed reunion with Nuit. In some rites of sexual magick, two magicians work together

---

Tibetan iconography is said to reflect the doctrine of active male and female passive wisdom. This is of course reversed in the Hindu Tantrik tradition where Kali is shown 'walking' on Shiva. 'Walking' on a love, is said to be sexual intercourse with the woman on top and therefore active whilst Shiva represents passive wisdom. Bharati acknowledges that the Tibetan posture has its problems if the man is meant to be the active partner.

adopting this god form.[8] One will assume the form of the overarching goddess Nuit shown in the picture and the other assumes the characteristic posture of Geb, the personification of the Earth[9]. This way of taking a technique from a magical picture strikes me as basically sound and I therefore suggest that it be extended to other glyphs in the Thelemic pantheon, more especially to the myth of the contendings of Seth and Horus.

The ancient Egyptian personification of Magick was Thoth. Thoth is a monstrous soul, he has the body of a man and the head of an ibis bird. There is an occult doctrine that says that knowledge can arise from the union of opposites such as human and beast. Thoth is often shown with the ibis head, a bird which according to Plutarch[10] taught humanity the therapeutic value of an enema. Thoth is also shown as an ape, a creature noted for its prodigious sexuality.

The way Thoth was said to have been born is magically significant. In one account Thoth miraculously springs from the head of Seth.[11] Seth was also born in a strange manner, bursting forth from the side of his mother Nuit. Miraculous birth must be a necessary prerequisite for any personification of Magick. This is a pattern that can be observed in other ancient cultures, for example in the Tibetan tradition the boddhisattva most closely associated with Magick is Padmasambhava, whose name means 'born from a lotus'.[12] In India the equivalent of Thoth could well be the elephant headed god Ganesha, who was moulded from the bodily secretions of his mother Parvati's skin. Shiva and Parvati represent everything that is unconscious in the human psyche writ large, and it is significant that they never produce their offspring or magical children by the conventional route.

---

8   This is a fairly common posture for sexual intercourse, whether ritual or not. Whether the gods taught it to humanity or the other way round is difficult to say.
9   Note that the personification of the Earth is not invariably female.
10 Plutarch *De Isis et Osirid*, ch 75.
11 J G Griffiths *The Contendings of Horus & Seth* (Liverpool UP 1960).
12 Yeshe Tsogyal, *The Lotus Born - the life story of Padmasambhava* (Shambala 1993)

As Brothers Fight Ye!

Sexuality amongst the ancient Egyptian Gods is an instructive area of study for the magician. There is at least one homosexual episode in which the participants are the Gods Seth and Horus. Seth lusted after his brother Horus. So Horus sought the advice of his mother Isis on how to avoid his brother's advances. Isis instructs Horus to submit to his brother but not to allow anal penetration to occur. Seth's semen is thereby caught between the fingers of Horus:

> Then Seth said to Horus, 'Come, let us spend a pleasant day in my house.' Horus replied to him 'Certainly, most certainly.' When the time of evening came, a bed was prepared for them and the two lay down. Now during the night Seth caused his penis to

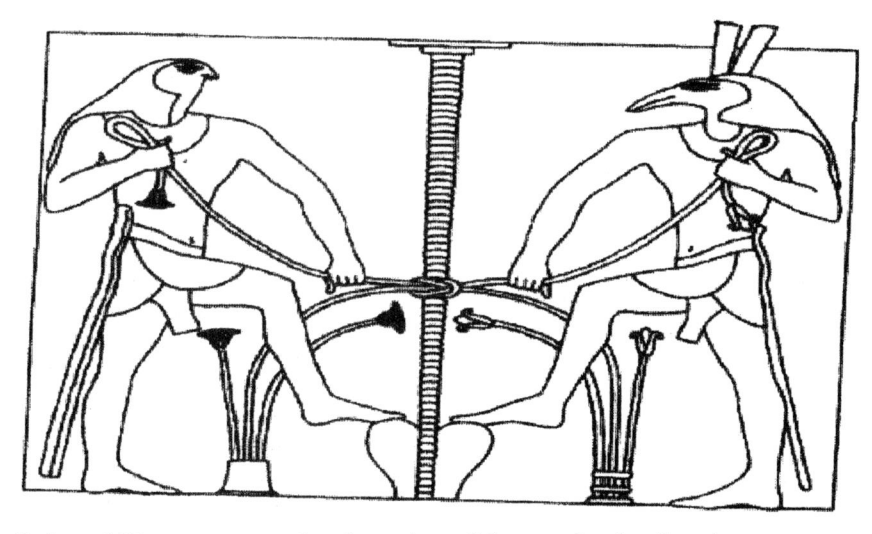

Seth and Horus representing the union of the two lands of ancient Egypt. Their feet rest upon lungs and windpipe, symbolising the breath or spirit.

As Brothers Fight Ye!

become erect and inserted it between the buttocks of Horus. And then Horus placed his two hands between his buttocks and took forth the semen of Seth'[13]. This he later sprinkled on Seth's favourite food, the lettuce, which incidentally is said to be an aphrodisiac.

This homosexual intercourse had been regarded as an isolated episode, of only subsidiary importance; but according to the author of one of the few useful books on the mythology of Seth, 'it forms an integral part and an indispensable link in the myth' of the contendings of Seth and Horus.[14] The conflict between Seth and Horus as recounted in the seventeenth chapter of the *Book Of The Dead* ends with the supposed castration of Seth and the blinding of Horus. However, H Te Velde suggests that the real meaning of this is that 'after Seth had withdrawn' his phallus from his close homosexual embrace with Horus, Horus' eye becomes small and loses its strength. The symbol of the Eye of Horus is probably too complex to recount here, but it is important to note that Horus regains his strength by seizing the testicles of Seth. This seizing has been mistaken for castration, but it may be that Seth's vital juices are empowered to rejuvenate and open the eye of Horus.

The other consequence of this homo-erotic episode in ancient Egypt was the birth of the Thoth, patron of magick. You will remember how Seth was tricked into eating his own semen and he then gave birth to Thoth. In another account, Thoth's birth is the result of another homosexual union between the ithyphallic[15] God *Min* and an enemy. Whoever his parents were, significantly no shame attached itself to Thoth by reason of the manner of his birth [16].

Crowley may well have known about the above piece of mythology and this may have influenced him to assume this god form

---

13 Terence Deakin 'Evidence for Homosexuality in Ancient Egypt' *International Journal of Greek Love* Vol 1 No 1 (NY 1965).
14 H Te Velde *Seth - God of Confusion* (Leiden, Brill 1967).
15 Meaning 'straight phallus' i.e. permanently erect god.
16 P Boylan *Thoth the Hermes of Egypt* (London 1922).

As Brothers Fight Ye!

along with Victor Neuburg during their so-called Paris Working. The first and arguably most successful of that series of workings was the invocation of Hermes, the Greek name for Thoth. At a crucial point in the ritual both priests intoned the mysterious 'Greek Couplet' which was composed for them by disciple and classical scholar Walter Duranty:

Jungitur in vati vates:[17]
rex inclyte rhabdou
Hermes tu venias, verba nefanda ferens

(The poet is united with the poet,
O Famous King of the Wand
Hermes! May you come bearing unpropitious words.)

By all accounts the ritual did not always go smoothly. Details in magical records of other sexual workings performed by Crowley make it clear that after orgasm the sexual secretions were imbibed as an elixir by one or both partners for Magical ends. It is unclear whether this practice was followed in the Paris Working but it seemed likely. There is of course no substantive reason why we shouldn't do a similar thing, although in these days of safe sex you may want to first treat the elixir by simple calcination, or reduction to ash.

There are plenty of example of calcination treatment within the magical tradition. For instance in the Hindu tantrik and medical tradition blood, semen, urine, and even faeces can be treasured parts of the pharmacopoeia. The *Rasaratnakara* describes the use of a smouldering pit of elephant's dung as a drying agent for some medicines.[18]. *Rasaratnakara* means 'making the jewel of rasa'. *Rasa* means gold and also the essence of the body's fluids and in India is synonymous with the practice of Alchemy. As Indian alchemy developed and made contact with its western neighbours, metallic

---

[17] 'Vate', is the term used by the Romans to describe one of the three classes of Celtic priests.
[18] (VIII 69-71).

As Brothers Fight Ye!

mercury became more and more important, and the old term 'rasa' was used to designate just the metallic variety, leaving out the reference to bodily fluids. However in Sanskrit the fact that the same word is used to designate bodily fluids and alchemical mercury means that there must be a fundamental unity of outlook.[19]

Historians of ancient Egypt tell us that as time passed they became progressively more xenophobic and hostile towards their neighbours. The god Seth seems to have become a victim of this process, and as a god of frontiers he was often associated with foreigners. Archaeologists have found very few traces of an actual Seth cult but presumably there once was one. Some spells have survived in the Graeco-Egyptian world, such as the following one addressed to the Typhon, the Greek term for Seth:

> As Typhon is the adversary of the sun
> even so inflame the heart and soul of
> Ammonius whom Helene bore[20]
> even so her own womb
> Adonai Abraxas Pinouti Sabaoth[21]
> Inflame the soul and heart of
> Ammonius whom Helene Bore
> Towards Serapiacus whom a slave-woman bore
> Now Now
> Quickly Quickly
> In this very hour
> In this very day
> Forthwith commingle the souls of them both
> And cause Ammonius himself whom Helene bore
> [to love] Serapiacus whom a slave-woman bore
> Every hour and every day and every night

---

19   Chris Morgan 'Catharsis' in *Celtic Dawn II* September 1988.
20   The entities that carry out a spell have to have accurate information about the ancestry of the participants.
21   These are what Crowley dubbed barbarous names and they are found in many similar spells including the fragment that forms the core of *Liber Samekh*.

As Brothers Fight Ye!

Dio Adonia
Most exalted of gods
Whose true name is Dioo and Adonia

This love spell was wrapped around a mud figure now lying in the Ashmolean museum, Oxford.[22] The use of a mud figure or mannequin to cast a spell is a remarkably old tradition, as this spell shows. Archaeologists tell us that Seth or Typhon was very commonly invoked in matters of the heart. This must surely be further evidence that Seth is a patron of non reproductive sex as opposed to other fertility deities like Osiris. The so-called 'Bornless One' ritual used so often by Crowley as a preliminary invocation is also an invocation of Seth and it also plays on many non-reproductive sexual themes.[23]

Egyptian mythology is still one of the most favoured traditions most favoured by magicians and the Egyptian, Coptic and Greek texts are perhaps the most profound and magical series of conjurations available. Advanced magick with these ideas could involve re-enactment of the primeval coupling described in ancient myths, accompanied by breaking of taboos. This can make Magick more potent and can lead more quickly to reintegration and liberation. The ancient Egyptian texts, which represent the very beginnings of magick significantly also validate homosexual magick between men, as in the Ashmolean spell, and between women, and in conjurations which, saying 'bind him or her', are specifically bisexual.

Seth is a complicated proposition. The symbolism of Seth and Horus relates to the unification of the two lands of Egypt (and the red and the white, as shown by their crowns), another symbol for the alchemical union. This union transcends the narrow confines of gender, flowing as it does from a more powerful polarity. Ambiguous Lord Seth is patron of all kinds of sexuality. To worship him men and women must throw off any rigid notions of what is or isn't natural.

---

22 A S Hunt 'An Incantation in the Ashmolean Museum' *Journal of Egyptian Archaeology* 15 1929 (p 155-157).
23 A Crowley *Magick in Theory and Practice* (RKP 1975).

As Brothers Fight Ye!

Seth, you are such a mystery to me,
just an impression a glimpse only
of what you were
all is destroyed,
but for the few traces,
some tracks
how was your worship done?
shall we ever know you?
prowling in the depth of the desert
the waste land
too frightening for us
Your seal flashes with power
the white edges now clear
the black fading into half-formed shapes
the head of Rameses
Seth, lord of confusion
ambiguous one
new aeon totem
Dearest Seth,
is our age now free and ready for your return?

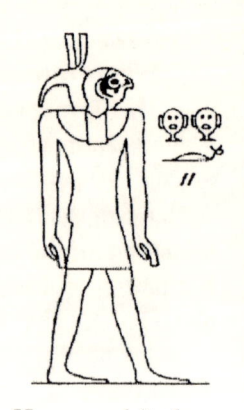

Horus and Seth united as 'he with the two faces'

You think that you live at a time when the old age is at last drawing to a close and a new one beginning. Only when the last vestiges of Victorianism are swept away will you be ready for any even more radical step; the integration of sexuality and spirituality. I wonder if the age of sexual repression is really over? You say that significant changes in the rules of sex have occurred in your lifetime. But these are not complete nor is it certain how abiding they will prove to be. I grant you that in all the long years of my exile never have there been such changes as those of the last few decades, they are spectacular. I do not take for granted some of the most radical changes in your race's history. Once again you may control your fertility through contraception and if necessary abortion. It is now as it was when I walked the earth. And the natural love between those of the same gender, this is no longer a crime punishable by stoning. The mysteries of the body are becoming known once again, sex is now a pleasure for women as it should be. And as the world was created by an act of self love so to is masturbation seen as a positive thing and not as self abuse. How I laughed when I read the prognostication of your so-called doctors, blaming self-love for the advent of all and any disease, when to the contrary it is the suppression of natural urges that leads to sickness, this all ancient physicians well knew. Even so, I feel a lingering paranoia, these changes may be temporary, mere aberrations in an unrelenting tapestry of repression.

You cannot lay the whole blame for this with Christianity. Is Christianity a hard machine like your industrial society or your economic system that places abstract laws of supply and demand above human emotions? Before the coming of the Christians the rot had started. It is difficult to believe there was ever a 'golden age' of pagan sexuality. The Christians merely continued a trend that was well started before them, they inherited the pagan tradition.[24] There are said to be 'three pillars' of western societies' sexual mores.

Intolerance of homosexuality; encouragement of indissoluble marriage; antagonism to pure sensual enjoyment; these were Greek and Roman virtues. Yes, I admit there were liberal trends but there was a backlash and this was called Stoicism. There were other, so-called ascetic doctrines, and they took hold just as Christianity was becoming a force. Roman law is the culprit and not Christian ethics. And you have been living under *pax romana* right up until your so-called industrial revolution. And Roman law, may I remind you, is hardly less repressive than the flesh-hating creed of Christianity

I shall give you an example. The Romans hated what they called 'passivity' especially in sexual encounters. Heterosexual or homosexual, it doesn't matter which, passivity is shameful. Only a slave could safely be passive, a perquisite of slavery you might say. But the Roman definition of passivity is perverse and included *excessive* sexual compliance in woman. In the city and in the

---

24 See Robin Lane Fox *Pagans and Christians* (Penguin)

As Brothers Fight Ye!

countryside a women was expected to discourage any sexual advantages, if only in token, even those of their husbands and lovers. Have you ever heard of anything more ridiculous?[25] And cunnilingus, the most wonderful of pleasures for a women and a man was thought shameful because it implied passivity! And the disciples of Sappho, they too were guilty of the sin of passivity. Little did those Roman moralists know.

The Roman moralist Seneca may have been a fool but he was an influential fool.[26] Marriages, so he thought, should not be based on love. The Christian monk Jerome or Saint Jerome, as the Christian prefer, merely echoes this when 'he cites the words of Sextus the Pythagorean, who says that a man who shows himself to be more violently in love with his wife than a husband (should be) is an adulterer . . . whereby a man should not treat his wife as if she were a harlot, not a woman her husband as if he were a lover, for the holy sacrament of marriage should be treated with all honour and reverence.'[27]

Pythagorus you know, was a bit of a prude. But we must not slander the Christians, they did manage to salvage one good idea. In the end they came round to the idea that love should in fact be the basis of marriage after all. They must be thanked for creating the only society that continued to subscribe to the novel ideal. It is perhaps one Christian idea we can keep whilst we must reject much other nonsense including indissoluble marriage.[28]

The pursuit of chastity, I hear you say, that must be a peculiarity of Christianity. Not so, the ideal of chastity was dreamt up by the ascetics and monks of the Stoic, Pythagorean and neo-Platonist variety.

---

25 Aries and Bejin (eds) *Western Sexuality: Practice and Precept in Past and Present Times* (Oxford 1986) p. 128.
26 Paul Veyne, 'Homosexuality in Ancient Rome' in Aries and Bejin *op cit.* p. 31
27 Quoted in Jean-Louise Flandrin 'Sex in married life in the Early Middle Ages' in Aries and Bejin *op cit.* p. 122
28 Luc Thore 'Language et Sexuality' in *Sexuality Humane* (Collection RES, Paris 1970) quoted in Aries and Bejin *op cit.* pp. 65-95.

As Brothers Fight Ye!

Personally I blame that serpent god Patanjali. He created yoga with his *Yogasutras* and the Greeks when they read it hadn't the wit to discern its true meaning. Chastity is indeed a form of mental control and non-attachment and if practised in moderation can have startling results for consciousness. However it should never have been applied to sexual ethics.[29]

Seth, you stand accused of sodomy, which is no longer a crime, at least not the homosexual variety.

That is a strange distinction.

Yes, by the sixteenth of our centuries, homosexual sodomy was a crime on a par with adultery. But even then the penalties for heterosexual sodomy were, if anything, more severe than for the homosexual variety, Even today, heterosexual sodomy remains, technically, a criminal offence. The Marquis de Sade believed that this was because the perpetrator was making a deliberate decision to avoid the 'proper' avenue of intercourse. But tell me Seth, are gay people then your chosen ones.

That depends on whether the medieval and ancient 'sodomite' is really the ancestor of the homosexual or gay. The sodomite is definitely of me, but I see that some of you say that the modern homosexual was not even born until Westphal wrote of him in 1870. Before that the sodomite was a sub species of criminal or even a separate human genus akin to androgyny. And your rap group *Public Enemy* says that there is no word in any African language for homosexual, boy have I got news for him, and I *know* Africa.[30]

But surely now, Seth, we live in less authoritarian times?

Is that some kind of joke? Even a few centuries ago, before your so-called industrial revolution, there were fewer sources of authority than today. When the main source of authority was the civil and canon law, it was *less* intrusive than the current proliferation of authorities. You are pulled every which way by the authority of the medical

---

29 Michel Foucault, 'The Battle for Chastity' in Aries and Bejin *op cit.*
30 See Randy Conner, *op cit.*

As Brothers Fight Ye!

establishment, still sometimes the church, the police, the judiciary, employers, social services and the educationalists.

Medieval authorities were simpler and focused on the family unit. Handbooks for use of church confessors recommend investigation in great detail of the activities of the family, including matrimonial sexuality. If you thought the inquisition was intrusive then the confessional will really surprise you. Questions were commonly asked concerning the position of intercourse, its frequency and the number and types of caress. You may like to think of this as an extension of the Inquisition but the parishioners themselves demanded such a dialogue. They wanted real information on sexual matters and who better to ask than for advice about sexual things than the clergy. There was a saying that 'no-one is happy after sex apart from dogs and clergy getting it for free.'

Sex was a dangerous business, a couple had to seek advice on what was and wasn't lawful behaviour. Marriages were still mainly arranged by matchmakers and the confessional might be the only source of marriage guidance counselling, unless you could read the classics. The so-called pagan philosopher Aristotle has a lot to answer for, he was obsessed with the economics of the sexual act. According to his theories, the male semen was the primary cause in reproduction and the female was of secondary importance, acting merely as a safe repository for the tiny baby contained in the semen. The medieval clergy, experienced as they were in sexual matters actually argued against the Aristotelian view, stating instead that the man and woman made equal contribution towards to development of a embryo. Thus in an age where inequality between the sexes was the almost invariably the norm, in theory and almost always in practice, the sexual exchange was perhaps the only exception. The clergy wrote this down in manual for use by other less experienced clergy.

I'll give you an example of the kind of things they wrote. Was the female 'semen' necessary for procreation? The female 'semen' was ejaculated at orgasm and a question arises concerning the consequences, moral and physical of lack of orgasm, a situation apparently not uncommon in this time.[31]

Another related question concerned whether it was lawful for the husband to prolong copulation until his wife had emitted her semen? And further was it desirable for the husband and wife to have an orgasm at the same time? Was it lawful for the wife to achieve orgasm by fondling herself after her husband had withdrawn, either as a form of contraception or because he had finished?

It is doubtful whether any of the above issues would have arisen in the Victorian confessional. Three or four centuries of industrial society had done much to throw a veil over sexuality. During this time there had also been widespread de-Christianization, if the rise in illegitimate births and pre-nuptial conception is anything to go by. Some have argued that industrial society needs reproduction but ideally without sexuality. A sensuous society may be less willing to rise before dawn and go to the factory. The zenith of this aspect of industrial society is Victorianism and many still feel its effects. Victorian society was highly paradoxical. It was able to place marriage on a pedestal whilst completely denying that women had any sexual side to their nature. It was a culture famous for the fact that some of its members veiled the legs of chairs and pianos because of their alleged lewdness and yet it had a very high rate of illegitimacy and a huge number of prostitutes. Brave souls such as Aleister Crowley sort to break out of the ignorant Victorian fog and there was a explosion of writing and talking about sex, but mainly confined to the scientific and therefore middle classes. The doctor scientist took on the traditional role of confessor and shaman. The Theosophist Annie Besant played a key role in the emancipation of women from sexual ignorance, although she was herself afflicted with the same ignorance of almost all Victorian women:

> I married in the winter of 1867 with no more idea of the marriage relation than if I had been four years old instead of twenty. My

---

[31] For a modern look at ancient doctrine of female ejaculation see: Josephine Lowndes Severly *Eve's Secrets* (London 1987)

As Brothers Fight Ye!

dreamy life, into which no knowledge of evil had been allowed to penetrate, in which I had been guarded from all pain, shielded from all anxiety, kept innocent on all questions of sex, was no preparation for married existence, and left me defenceless to face the rude awakening. Looking back on it all, I deliberately say that no more fatal blunder can be made that to train a girl to womanhood in ignorance of all life's duties and burdens and then let her face them for the first time away from all old associations . . . That 'perfect innocence' may be very beautiful, but it is a perilous possession and Eve should have the knowledge of good and evil ere she wanders forth from the paradise of a mother's love.

Many an unhappy marriage dates from its very beginning, from the terrible shock to a young girl's sensitive modesty and pride, her helpless bewilderment and fear.

Men with their public school and college education, or knowledge that comes by living in the outside world, may find it hard to realise the possibility of such infantile ignorance in many girls. Nonetheless, such ignorance is a fact in the case of some girls at least, and no mother should let her daughter, blindfold, slip her neck under the marriage yoke.[32]

Only in this century have things really changed for the better, at least as far as the people of the metropolis. But as we approach the millennium it is far from clear what the outcome will be. The forces of reaction, fundamentalism of all kinds, Hindu, Islamic and Christian, are trying to force sex back into the closet. By understanding how this happened in the past we can resist them. Experience and history shows the greatest danger you face comes from the restriction of ideas not from their liberation. As your prophet Wilhelm Reich succinctly put it, an emotional plague is our greatest threat and this time we must not let it prevail.

Seth, Lord of Confusion and ambiguity,

---

32   Annie Besant *An Autobiography* (London 1895) p. 71

As Brothers Fight Ye!
teach us more of your purpose in this age of rebirth and change.

Your scientists say that of all aspects of human physiology, the best understood is called endocrinology - literally the science of the internal web or internal network of glands that regulate the creation, growth, and maintenance of the human organism. The endocrine system has proved a fascination for occultists, especially those with an interest in sexual magick and the Tantrik psychic anatomy of the six chakras.

The endocrine system does much to determine who we are; through it we can receive our true gender. At the risk of asking the obvious, I put it to you, is there such a thing as a true gender?

Your poet Alexander Pope wrote in *The Rape of the Lock*

For spirits freed from mortal laws, with ease,
Assume what sexes and what shapes they please.

This is a very old truth indeed, but your modern philosophers are only now asking the same questions:

'do we truly need a true sex? With a persistence that borders on stubbornness modern western societies have answered in the affirmative. They have obstinately brought into play this question of a true sex in an order of things where one might have imagined that all that counted was the reality of the body and the intensity of its pleasure.'[33]

In the nineteenth century the existence of the hermaphrodite had become a medieval myth. It was deemed impossible for two genders to reside in one person. Two basic genders, male and female, was all that is possible. But even a cursory look at your own DNA shows this to be a mistaken view. Human beings have forty-sex chromosomes consisting of twenty three identical pairs; one half of the pair is

---

33 Michel Foucault, *Herculine Barbine: being the recently discovered memoirs of a nineteenth century French hermaphrodite* (Harvester 1980) p. vii.

As Brothers Fight Ye!

contributed by each parent. Deviations in this array often do occur and they result in some quite gross physical deviations from the so-called norm. Some of these so-called deviations only come to light by chance for they do not invariably effect the ability of the bearer to lead a 'normal' life, whatever that might mean. Many of you possess abnormalities in your chromosomes that have gone undetected, you will probably never know how many of you are really 'normal'.[34]

According to this same chromosomal theory sexual differentiation is determined by one pair of genes on one pair of chromosomes, the so-called sex chromosomes. In sexual reproduction the mother contributes a female chromosome which is labelled X and the father contributes *either* a male *or* a female chromosome which is labelled X or Y. I draw the conclusion from this that men have an ambiguous gender or are deep down androgynous.

If you look at the way the sex chromosomes combine in sexual reproduction some of the implications of this may become clearer.

XXX In this permutation one of the parents has contributed two female chromosomes (XX) and the other one chromosome (X), making an usual configuration of XXX, the so-called hyper-female. Very little is known about the incidence of this type in the general population. Charlotte Wolff, who in her day was a respected sexologist, said such women were sterile and mentally retarded although thus is not confirmed by other authorities and it may be an unwarranted generalisation.[35]

XYY. Just as there is a so-called hyper-female, there is, at the other end of the spectrum, a so-called hyper-male. These men combine one female chromosome from one parent with two male chromosomes from the other. More is known about the hyper-male than the hyper-female as there have been several studies of them, but mainly amongst prison populations and this may invalidate some of the findings. The

---

34 Ronald Flescher *Lecture Notes on Endocrinology* (Blackwell Scientific)
35 Charlotte Wolff *Bisexuality* (Quartet)

XYY male is said to be excessively tall and masculine.[36] Some of the ideas about the XYY type are a bit suspect.

So the hyper-male and hyper-female do not rule the earth. The commonest type, nearly fifty percent of the population of apparently characteristic (phenotype) females or males have just two sex chromosomes, either XX or XY. There has been some discussion amongst occultists whether the female XX is the basic chromosomal type or whether that position belongs to the male XY type. There is even a bizarre discussion of which came first, the goddess or the god, the issue being decided on the basis of biological differences as those outlined above. On the face of it, *logic* would seem to say that XY (the male) must come before XX (female). However some commentators have argued that all embryos' 'prototypes', *look* like females until transformed by hormones secreted by the mother, which causes some of them to mutate into males. If biological determinism is important to you, perhaps these facts are important.

The Third Sex

I would remind you, that almost all ancient cultures, including the ancient Egyptian, recognised three genders, he, she and it and furthermore they almost all concur that the first human being was male *and* female. Your own science of genetics has vindicated the ancient view. This gender is closest to my own heart, the third one (XX,XY). I even took the form of a god for my Greek lovers who knew me as Hermaphrodite.[37] I combined Hermes and Aphrodite. My follower Theoprastus (482-287 BC), gave the world one of the first descriptions of Hermaphroditus. Heroditus also recounts the story that the Scythians were hermaphrodites and as a consequence possessed supernatural powers taught to them by Aphrodite. Even Plato could not resist writing of me in his *Symposium*. There are several rare statues to

---

36 I once spoke to a male to female transexual who claimed to be a XYY male.
37 Marie Delacourt, *Hermaphodite* (London)

be seen in the world's great museums, including the Vatican. They fall into two main types. There are those that are purely symbolic and are unlikely to have any human incarnations. These are recognisable by the fact that the male/female split is ranged either side of the body's mid line. Thus the left is female and the right male. This, according to your own biological theory, is not the way hermaphroditism actually presents itself. However, other images of Hermaphrodite show a more regular combination of male and female sexual characteristics. The best is of a beautiful young woman who is raising her dress to expose her genitals. This ritual act serves to expose the normal female vulva but with an erect phallus projecting upwards. (It is normal for such statutes to be turned towards the wall in the more prudish galleries.)

Hermaphrodite does indeed have human incarnations. Although rare about one thousand cases have been described, mainly in medical literature. During the nineteen century, the medical profession began to doubt my existence but this has now been confirmed by modern endocrinology. According to modern clinical belief, the chromosomes are a simple doubling of the standard type. That is to say, the 'true' hermaphrodite has two pairs of sexual chromosomes, XX,XY or XX,XXY being the most common.

At one time known hermaphrodites were called as criminals. In the middle ages it was acknowledged that two sexes could reside in one body but the law demanded that the godfather nominate a sex for the raising of the child until adulthood. Thereafter the hermaphrodite could choose to remain in that sex or change it and even to marry. The hermaphrodite could not change their mind again and if they did, (which presumably they did or why legislate?) the law might accuse them of sodomy, a capital offence. In the age of clinical medicine, the hermaphrodite lost this freedom of choice which was exercised on his or her behalf by a doctor at birth. I wonder why this was felt necessary, perhaps a fear of any ambiguity was a feature of the industrial age. Indeed it was just such a fear of the ambiguous that was successfully played upon by many Surrealists, most famously Marcel Duchamp who adopted the female gender as a way of completely overturning his given personality. The magical power of ambiguity has

As Brothers Fight Ye!

exercised many great minds.[38] The magicians Aleister Crowley and Austin Osman Spare were both fascinated with Hermaphrodite, nothing surprising there perhaps. There is an interesting autobiography of a hermaphrodite who went under the name Herculine Barbine, which is worth a read.

My ancestor, the divine Akhanaten, who composed several of the hymns in the *Old Testament* 'Book of Psalms', (although strangely they are credited to some nonentity called David!) may have been a hermaphrodite or something similar. Some of your scientists claim he was an XXY male and may have been suffering from *Klinefelter's* syndrome. The joke is that it didn't seem to have affected his fertility and he fathered several children, including Tutankhamun.

I'm only telling you all this because I want you to realise that gender is not a simple matter. Even at the level of basic mechanistic biology it is possible to see some variation from the simplistic model of two genders. To be either male or female is not the most important thing. The point of the above discussion was to show how some of you can never categorically affirm I am just a man or just a woman. Your biology, thought pathological by the doctors of your age, will not allow it. But the normal majority have no reason for complacency either. Apart from when reproducing, an activity which takes but a small part of your life, most of you are either physically or psychically part of the third, most numerous, gender. The pagan view is based on a pantheon of gods that are reflected in the human population. The gods are many genders and every gender and physical type, as are you. Some gods are especially connected with the pleasures and pain of sexuality. Realisation of your basic amorphous, bisexual nature is a source of real magical power, this is the true meaning of the mysteries of Seth, which I have returned in order to teach.

---

38 Mary Douglas *Purity and Danger* (RKP 1978)

Chapter 4
The Erotic Landscape

Magicians have always had a well-developed sense of *spirit of place*. Some places have a magical feel to them, and are natural places to work magick or merely to go for the magical equivalent of a quest or pilgrimage. The travelling through a magical or erotic landscape is something that has re-emerged into modern magick during the last two decades. But this sense of the holy being attached to particular places was also a distinguishing feature of the ancient Indo-Europeans, pagan Celts at one extreme or ancient Indians at the other. Pilgrimage in India is said to be non-Aryan in origin, that is to say it can be traced to indigenous tribal roots[1]. The orthodox religions of today, whether Hindu, Muslim or Christian were originally hostile to such ideas, which they thought smacked of primitive animism and magick. However the power of the landscape won through and the desire for pilgrimage re-emerged to become an important feature of even these hidebound creeds. By way of 'revenge' tantrik elements subvert the

---

[1] A Bharati, 'Pilgrimage in the Indian Tradition' *Journal of the History of Religions* (University of Chicago 1963) p. 149.

The Erotic Landscape

more orthodox pilgrimage, as at the famous Jaganath festival, where the offering (prasad) given to pilgrims is secretly sprinkled with wine.[2]

The making of a regular pilgrimages to sacred spots is still an important duty for many of the world's devotees and one which earned a great deal of personal merit. For example Mecca, the birthplace of the prophet Mohammed is the chief destination of Muslim pilgrimage. At Mecca the pilgrim finds the 'Kaaba', a huge tented area forbidden to non-Muslims. The Kaaba is a large black megalith thought originally to be a meteorite. It seems strange to me that a religion like Islam should have such a geomantic heart comparable to the 'omphalos' of the Celts and Indo-Europeans. In every mosque is a niche or slab called a Mihrab which indicates the direction of Mecca. This direction, also known as the Kiblah, is the point to which all mosques are oriented throughout the world.

Second in fame only to Mecca must be the river Ganges. All Hindus would hope to visit the Ganges at least once in their lifetime and to die there if possible; something only a relatively tiny percentage would ever manage.

In the Christian tradition the focus is the Holy Land, the birth place of their saviour Jesus and Jerusalem, the place of his final apotheosis. In medieval times, when pilgrimage was at it most valued, if you couldn't get to the holy land, a far-off town might be deemed to be a symbolic equivalent. For example Rocamadour in Southern France, has a processional or initiatory way, which follows the stations of the cross. Closer to home, one may use a particular saint's resting place, venerated by tales of that person's own travels in distant lands or even a mere fragment of their body, held as a relic.

In tantrism there is also a keen sense of spirit of place. Tantriks call their sacred sites *Pitha*, which distinguishes them from orthodox Hindus who use the totally different term - *tirtha*. The tantrik pithas[3]

---

[2] Bharati (1963).
[3] The classic work on pithas is still S C Sircar's 'The Sakta Pithas', *Journal of the Royal Asiatic Society* (Bengal) Vol XIV 1948 pp. 1-108.

always designate a shrine of the primal goddess.[4] For example in a very old tantrik text of my own (Nath) tradition, it is a place of pilgrimage as well as somewhere to sit and meditate.[5] Pitha, which means 'seat' is also a piece of tantrik *twilight* language and is a euphemism for 'yoni'.

These same ancient texts tell us that there are four most important Pithas or pilgrimage sites, although sometimes a few others are added, making the total up to seven; sometimes one hundred and eight are mentioned, an especially auspicious number in this tradition; and sometimes they are said to be countless.

The origin of these pilgrimage sites is the matter of legend, and the details of this legend make it clear we are dealing with an eternal or archetypal myth; one that recurs in several other cultures of the Indo-European heritage and even outside of it. This may be called *the* tantrik myth and revolves around the story of Sati, consort of Shiva and personification of the goddess. Shiva and Sati have retired to their mountain paradise. meanwhile Sati's father Daksa (whose name means 'ritual skill') plans a great sacrifice, to which he invites all divine beings with the exception of Shiva and his wife. Daksa plans this insult to Shiva because he does not approve of his alliance with his daughter and may even harbour incestuous desires for Sati. But the insult is too much for Sati to bear and she kills herself, in some versions, by flinging herself onto the sacrificial fire, thus giving her name to the subsequent practice of widow self-sacrifice. When Shiva eventually arrives on the scene he kills Daksa and destroys the feast, engendering

---

[4] This information comes from A Bharati, (1970), but he also supplies an interesting counter example when he describes *Dattatreyapitha*, a hill sacred to the tantrik guru Dattatreya. located near Mysore (Chikmaghlur district) although over the years the guru/guardianship of the shrine has passed into Muslim hands. p. 186.

[5] P C Bagchi (ed) *Kaulajnana Nirnaya* translated into English by Mike Magee (Prachya Prakashan 1987).

The Erotic Landscape

many new human diseases.[6] This part of the myth is very old, the oldest version traceable to the ancient *Rig Veda* and it may well be older than that.

In medieval India, at the time when tantrism was at its height, this myth was again embellished. Shiva was too late to save Sati but he discovers the remains of her body. He picks her up and sobbing with grief, carries her about the universe. Eventually the god Vishnu is called upon to end this potentially disruptive situation. He follows Shiva, gradually slicing up the body of Sati. The four most magically potent pieces of her body fall to the ground and give rise to the four[7] most sacred places or pithas of tantrism.[8] These are her genitals, nipples and tongue.[9]

The earliest reference to four principal tantrik pilgrimage centres or pithas occurs in the seventh century of our era. It may well be Buddhist in origin. The Sahajayana sect of Buddhism, was distinguished by the doctrine that eternal bliss can arise from sexual pleasure and that the Buddha in the form of Vajrasattva had ritual intercourse with yoginis in four sacred places or seats. In the Hindu tantrik tradition the first pitha is the only one still currently active and is at Kamarupa in Assam. As its name suggests, it is the place where the yoni of the goddess fell. This site has seven lesser (upa) pithas, where dwell the seven siddhas or powerful ones. Kamarupa represents

---

[6] See Kris Morgan, *Medicine of the Gods* (Mandrake of Oxford 1994) p. 64

[7] There are accounts of 108 seats of the goddess, in some the cult object is a representation of the severed limb. In Bharati (1963) p. 167 he describes the shrine of Mukhambika - mouth mother at Connamore on the Malabar coast. It shows the lower part of the head only, and in a nearby shrine is the Golden Mother, which is depicted as a pair of golden hands reaching out of a well.

[8] David Kinsley *Hindu Goddesses* (University of California Press 1986).

[9] There is an early version of this myth recorded in the *Mahabharata* XII 282-3

the eastern quarter. The second pitha is known as Purnagiri; it lies in the south, its actual location undecided, and represents the left nipple or sometimes the navel. The third pitha is Uddiyana (the garden), situated in north-west India, in Kashmir, and can be attributed to the right nipple or sometimes the throat. Uddiyana is also the name of an important Bandha used to control the vital breath. The fourth is Arvudama, in Jalandhara in East Punjab, representing the tongue. An earlier tradition may have had three basic sites.[10]

Bharati suggests that 'the association of the limbs of the sadhaka, or magician, with certain localities may have given rise to the belief regarding particular limbs of the mother goddess.'[11] A characteristic feature of tantrik rites is the use of the hands to energize parts of the body by 'installing' corresponding images of gods and goddesses, whilst intoning the appropriate power mantra. The name for this technique is *nyasa*.

Sircar hints that the section of the myth added by the medieval tantriks was Greek or Egyptian in origin. I have spoken much of the migration of ideas from India to the west into Europe and beyond, and east into China. But this transmission went two ways. This is most obvious when you look at the history of astrology in India, which is clearly derived from Greek, Babylonian and Egyptian sources.[12] The myth of the murder and dismembering of the God Osiris by Seth is one that could have been known in India from Greek sources. The sacred cult centres of ancient Egypt are reputed to have originated in this act, as Isis traversed the landscape searching for the discarded limbs of her beloved Osiris; the phallus was lost for ever, eaten by the Oxyrhynchus fish, the oasis of Oxyrhynchus being a cult centre of the God Seth.

---

[10] There are of course many more than four pithas and the canonical tantrik text is the *Mahapitha Purana* which lists the traditional sacred number of 108.
[11] Bharati, (1963) p. 149
[12] See David Pingree 'History of Mathematical Astronomy in India' *Dictionary of Scientific Biography*, Vol 15, supp.1 (Scribners 1978)

The Erotic Landscape

The Egyptian myth of the Oxyrhynchus fish is a close parallel to a tantrik story, of a scroll containing forbidden knowledge. In the Indian tradition this was swallowed by a fish, or sometimes overheard by a human temporarily transformed into a fish, which amounts to the same thing. The fish is eventually caught and the scroll discovered by a fisherman. This fisherman is to be Matsyendranath, the first guru of the Nath sect of Hindu tantriks.

Buddhism was one of the first religions to develop a lively cult of relic worship, which we should distinguish from the notion of spirit of place. The Buddhist stupa is in fact a structure designed to encase relics.[13] Some anthropologists believe that myths of dismemberment are remnants of the ancient practice of animal and human sacrifice. Indeed, tantrik ideas are often traceable to non-Aryan tribal groups that worshipped fierce aspects of the goddess often with bloody sacrifice. The influx of archaic pagan ideas lies at the heart of even the most orthodox of religions. For instance, in medieval Europe, pieces of the body of a saint were kept and venerated at almost every important cult centre; in fact this was what often made them important. Glastonbury in Wiltshire was a focus on this score because of the legend that Joseph of Arimathea brought two vials of blood and clear fluid, supposed to be the blood of the Christian God. Of course this practice was often satirised as in Chaucer's *Pardoner's Tale*, where the pardoner had sold enough pieces of the *true* cross to build an ark! The history of religions provides evidence of the gradual abolition of human and later animal sacrifice. In ancient times, the biblical story of Abraham's instruction to sacrifice his son (Gen.20.22), is good example of this discourse. Perhaps the rite of circumcision is a replacement of the more archaic and brutal practice. In almost every culture blood sacrifice was given a purely symbolic gloss, although until at least the nineteenth century the thuggees, particularly brutal devotees of the goddess Kali, initiated a revival of human sacrifice, and some reports tell of its periodic outbreak even in the present day.

---

[13] Bharati (1963) p. 152

Sexual Magick

The myth of the dismembered goddess accounts for the presence in the Indian landscape of a number of pilgrimage sites sacred to her. There is also a myth to account for the male sacred sites, and the focus for this is the lingam or phallus of Lord Shiva. It is tempting to believe that the mythology of Shiva and his first and second wife, accounts for a great deal of Indian geomancy. Shiva loses his lingam in a conflict with Vishnu, itself very reminiscent of the conflict of Seth and Horus described in chapter three. Shiva is able to reconstitute his own lingam, which is just as well as the same fate befalls him several times. The discarded lingams are venerated, according to tradition, at twelve places throughout India. One of these is at Grishneshwar, in Maharashtra, close to one of the wonders of the world at Ellora. Another of these is an Ice-lingam situated in the Himalayas. The lingam is Shiva, and many of its features are what this god personifies; sexuality in itself often opposed to fertility; the power of expansion that in some myths is infinite, symbolising the power of the phallus to create ad infinitum.

So far we have described the genesis of 'male' and 'female' points in the landscape. The question arises now as to how one would recognise such places. To the mystic gaze, the landscape has an erotic quality, almost any tall phallus shaped rock would be sacred to Lord Shiva, whilst the more rounded hills, and rivers or streams are almost always sacred to a goddess. It is not necessarily for the feature to be as large as a hill in order for it to evoke this feeling in the devotee. Numerous temples in India are built over quite small pieces of rock, no more than a few feet in height or length. These again are often either phallic shaped stones, occurring naturally and termed jyoti-lingams; or flat slabs, often dredged out of river beds. There is a fine example of this at a place called Amber, just outside of Jaipur in Rajasthan. In the temple to Kali is an image of Sila Devi, a perfect black slab. The goddess appeared to the Maharaja Man Singh in this form and granted him the boon of parenthood. The slab was transported to the fort and a white marble temple built closed by solid silver doors, embellished with twenty aspects of Kali. The temple is oriented to the north which is a

The Erotic Landscape

common feature of Kali temples and in striking contrast to other cults where the image is oriented towards the east.

Hindu temple architecture is completely permeated by geomantic ideas. The basic ground plan of a temple is a stylised picture of the human form called a mandala. A temple is therefore commensurate with a living organism and the holy of holies is called a *garbha*, literally a womb or vagina.

All these ideas have parallels in our own European tradition. One need look no further than Glastonbury, thought by some to be a major nexus of earth energy within Britain. The site is much more complex than the famous Tor, which is only the male/phallic counterpart to the more rounded Chalice Hill a few hundred yards away. This feminine, almost breast like hill yields a beautiful sacred spring of iron-rich and red tinged water from the Chalice Well gardens at its base and in the valley between the two inclines. The motif of the disembodied phallus is also recalled by the countless legends in this country of the devil dropping parts of his body, or sometimes a rock he happened to be carrying at the time.

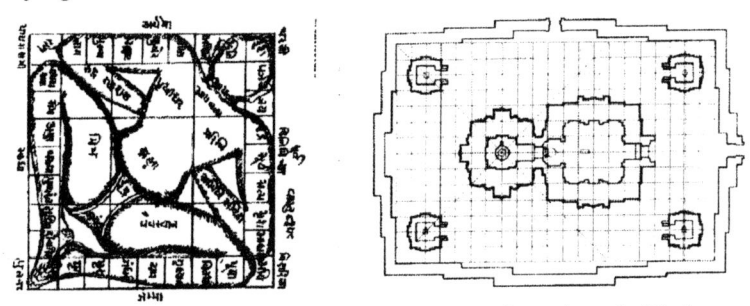

Left: Correspondence between human body and floor plan of a Hindu temple, from an old architectural manual.
Right: Grid plan of a basic Hindu temple.

Sexual Magick

The cult of the elephant headed deity, Ganesha, the child part of the holy tantrik family of Shiva and Parvati has its main stamping ground and cult centre in Maharashtra. In that state there are eight main shrines to Ganesha; eight is appropriate as he is the Indian Thoth or Hermes. They are arranged over hundreds of miles to form a mandala and processional route. The pilgrim visits the so-called *Astavinayaka* (remover of obstacles) shrines. All eight contain self-existent images (svayambhu) that are said to have appeared to devotees in the form of elephant headed stones. The pilgrimage of all eight shrines constitutes a circumambulation of the boundaries of the sacred cosmos that is permeated by the presence of Ganesha. Circumambulation is a very ancient form of worship which may have its origin in solar worship.[14] Ganesha is of course the son of Shiva and therefore a popular extension of the tantrik pantheon. It is mainly in the tantrik tradition that we find this element of worship of natural features of the land associated with the breasts, the generative organs or a natural rock suggestive of the deity. Tantrism is rooted 'in the low castes of India, or outside the orthodox pale. Many of its features are survivals of ancient religious folklore. It may represent the final stage of a vegetation festival, where the use of drugs and alcohol and breaking of erotic taboos were much used in agrarian rituals.'

One might be wondering what relevance this can have for you - unless one is able to visit these sites, it all seems a bit academic. Here paradoxically one has a point of contact with the tantrik. India is a big country, and for most tantriks, the making of a pilgrimage is out of the question, except perhaps as a once in a lifetime event. In fact it might be said that it is easier for a westerner to visit India than it is for an Indian tantrik to pilgrimage. There are two alternatives - firstly, to look for equivalent sacred spots nearer to home, and secondly, to internalise the pilgrimage into an internal journey through one's own body.

The finding of a corresponding sacred site for pilgrimage is a common feature of religious experience. You don't have to swallow

---

[14] Circumambulation = Sanskrit *pradakshina*, Although Bharati (1970) thinks that tantrik rites have less circumambulation.

The Erotic Landscape

banal explanations of the phenomenon where a supposed sacred site is merely a local tourist attraction. Esoterically it indicates that the would-be pilgrim has developed a feel for that particular archetype. As in the Ganesha shrines already mentioned, and indeed all of the Shiva and Shakti shrines, they arose because a devotee had attuned him or herself properly and could see the force in a stone or in the landscape. In the case of river shrines, the most celebrated river for pilgrimage is the Ganges and after that the Jamuna. The devotee naturally sees an aspect of the river goddess in the local tributary, just as the tantrik comes to see the primeval Goddess or God in a particular person, or best of all in the generative parts of that person. Confluences of rivers were particularly sacred in ancient India, and indeed today it may be worth looking for undiscovered sacred places at forgotten confluences in your own locality. Abodes of gods, magicians or philosophers are also important magical places and there are plenty of those in Europe, for instance Mount Olympus or Boleskine.

Tantrik thought is characterised by its anthropocentrism, that is, the fact that it places, accurately so I think, the human being at the centre of the universe: 'Here (within this body) is the Ganges, and the Jumna, here is Prayaga and Banares, here the sun and moon. Here the sacred places, here the Pithas and the Upa Pithas. I have not seen a place of Pilgrimage and abode of Bliss like my body.'

A second important alternative to physical pilgrimage is the internal variety developed and widely used by tantrik magicians. As Mircea Eliade put it in *Yoga, Immorality and Freedom*, the tantriks absorbed and systematised certain cosmic/natural ideas, so that they become reified within the body. Later on the same ideas are re-imposed on nature with startling effects. The human body corresponds to and is even identical with the universe. The body is often described as the cosmic mount Meru - the axis mundi or even as a tree, whose seed is to be found in the heart. The details of all this are too many and complicated - as is indeed the world - to go into here but the principle is an absolutely crucial one for the tantrik whose ritual almost always makes use of this image which is installed within the body by ritual gestures (*nyasa*). The most widely known version is found in Kundalini

Sexual Magick

Yoga; although I say widely known, but it is remarkable how often this well documented system is completely misunderstood. The central Nadi or yogic duct 'susumna' is to be likened to the world mountain; the two lateral ducts at the left and right (Ida and Pingala) to sacred rivers. Ida, which according to the *Kularnava Tantra* (15.35ff) connects with the lunar number sixteen and is the Ganges. Pingala, according to the same source, connects with the solar number twelve and represents the Yamuna river. Incidentally tantrik numerology is based on counting the number of syllables in a word or mantra. The celebrated Shrividya mantra should also have sixteen syllables.

A member of a tantrik sect in this country, of which there are a small dedicated band, would naturally have a veneration for the land, which is interposed with his or her own body. It is completely within the parameters of the tantrik tradition to search for the sites within the local geography that correspond to the places or chakras within the body. Flowing around these are the sacred rivers, such as the river Isis or Thames, a name derived from the Celtic term Tamesis or Tafwys, which may well be its titular goddess. Local holy wells, the 'digits' of that river along with suitable phallic sites help complete the sacred geography. It remains to worship the Earth Goddess, in her local form. That the worship of local genii was part of the tantrik tradition, as elsewhere in the Indo-European world, is established by the fact that so many names for gods and goddess are used in ancient texts.

Once the sacred geometry is discovered, the location is alive and vibrant - as are the devotees. In ritual magicians re-enact the primal dismemberment of the god or goddess. One person may touch or install the appropriate aspects of that divinity into another's body. This can be done by focusing first on your own body, becoming aware or visualising the appropriate god forms. For instance in the region of the heart resides your titular or self-chosen (*istadevata*) deity. You can use the breath to awaken and release them and transport the deity out of your body via the nostrils where it is placed onto a mandala or someone's body. This technique can be used to consecrate the body, limb by limb until the whole is a living mandala. There is little need to enumerate all the correspondences here, this can be created afresh or

The Erotic Landscape

gleaned from many of the books already mentioned. When the installation is complete it is appropriate to worship the Mandala and lovemaking is thought by tantriks to be a particularly appropriate form of worship.

A task for a ritual group or individual is to find as much as possible about local history and the locations of sacred sites, especially streams and springs which are the most vulnerable to destruction, often as not by Christians. By the practice of tantrik yoga you can undergo an internal and external circumambulation of these sites, revivifying both the landscape and yourself. These places can in turn be viewed as part of an even greater cosmological pattern of sacred geometry stretching through the whole of this land and beyond. When the scattered parts of the gods are reassembled we shall indeed be lifted up out of individual egos and become part of a greater reality of the erotic land.

Appendix One
Woman To Woman

(The following is the text of a letter received in response to the original publication of the first chapter. It was published in *NUIT-ISIS* #3 Autumn Equinox issue 1987)

I write to say how much I enjoyed reading the article by Katon Shual on the subject of Sexual Politics and Sexual Magick. I was particularly inspired by the section on homosexuality and thought it refreshing not to say brave of him to tackle the issue. This was something never before encountered in any similar magazine, especially the mention of lesbianism, on which there was a total silence until your piece, apart from those journals that stem from the separatist/feminist movement.

I share the author's contention that it is absurd to view the sexual act as something divorced from the emotions and feelings. Occultists often write as if sex is just another technique and the finding of a magical partner comparable to the finding of just another magical instrument or device. I also find it absurd that heterosexuality is somehow held up as 'superior' to an act of love between two people of the same sex. Perhaps many magicians have forgotten what love in sex is, in their pursuit of magical power and results.

I speak as someone who was involved with men both as sexual and magical partners for many years. I now live with a woman with whom I have a very close and also magically potent relationship.

Appendix one

There is a great deal of discussion on the occult scene of polarity. Polarity is used in rather a vague way, in the same way as 'ley-lines'. In my experience polarity is more to do with aspect than gender. It is therefore ridiculous to think that merely placing a man next to a woman in a ritual is going to produce a natural polarity. Done like this it is hit or miss whether things will click. And even if some energy does flow, one still runs the age old risk of establishing a flow of energy that is one-sided.

It seems that generally the criticism against female/female polarity working is that it will produce an inner imbalance. This view is founded upon a misconception that needs to be destroyed. This is that what is female equates with what is Yin, passive, 'negative' and what is Yang, active, 'positive' and solar. Even the briefest glimpse at Egyptian mythology will explode this simplistic yet generally held magical belief. Thoth is a moon God, Sekhmet a fire/sun Goddess and Isis is an archetype of the complete woman, wearing the sun-disk 'cloaked with the stars', of the moon and water, rising from the earth.

If sexual magick is partly used to produce an inner balance it is thus equally valid for a priestess of one aspect to work opposite a priestess of another. For example, a solar priestess can polarize with an earth or lunar priestess, a stellar priestess can work opposite an earth priestess etc. Two women can interchange these aspects in a very subtle and powerful way, relating to seasonal changes etc. Women have the added polaric interchange between 'dark and light' aspects of the menstrual cycle. The magical interchange between two women is potentially therefore extremely rich and very valid. It is about time that women broke out of this limited magical role as only lunar priestesses.

In conclusion is seems to me important for women to work together in the above way. And it goes to say that men should also not hesitate to work together on these lines if the feeling is there. All of this can only compliment the work of those involved with the heterosexual current. The reason why we practise this magick is a whole new topic not to be discussed here. But in a sentence, we are all striving to discover the subtleties and potentials of our own nature, limited as it once was by traditional expectations.   Julie Hayes Leeds

Bibliography

Aries P and Bejin A (eds) *Western Sexuality: Practice and Precept in Past and Present Times* (Oxford 1986).

Baring-Gould Sabine, *Curious Myths of the Middle Ages* (Jupiter Books 1977).

Berridge, Edward 'Respiro' *The Brotherhood of the New Life, or The Man, The Seer, The Adept, The Avatar, or T Lake-Harris, the Inspired Messenger* (Allen 1897).

Besant Annie, *An Autobiography* (London 1895).

Bharati, A., 'Pilgrimage in the Indian Tradition' *Journal of the History of Religions* (University of Chicago 1963)

Bharati., A., *The Tantric Tradition* (Rider 1970).

Bible, RSV version.

Bose, M., *The Post Caitanya Sahajiva Cult of Bengal* (Calcutta 1938)

Boylan P., *Thoth the Hermes of Egypt* (London 1922).

Charaka Samhita, English translation by Sharma and Dash, (Chowkhamba 1977)

Colquhoun Ithell, *The Sword of Wisdom - MacGregor Mathers and The Golden Dawn* (Spearman 1975).

Conner, Randy, *Blossom of Bone - reclaiming the connections between homoeroticism and the sacred* (Harper Collins 1993)

Corbin, Henry, 'L'Imago Templi', *Spring* Vol 43 (1974); 'La Configuration du Temple de la Ka'ba comme secret de la vie spirituelle' Spring, Vol 34 (1965). Both these articles are in English and are reprinted in his *Eranos-Jahrbuch*.

Crowley Aleister, *The Confessions of Aleister Crowley - An Autohagiography* edited by John Symonds & Kenneth Grant (London, Cape 1969)

Crowley Aleister, *Magick* (RKP 1972)

Daniélou, Alain, *Shiva and Dionysus*, reprinted as *Gods of Love and Ecstasy* (Inner Traditions 1992)

Dasgupta's *Obscure Religous Cults as background of Bengali Literature*, (Calcutta 1946)

Deakin Terence, 'Evidence for Homosexuality in Ancient Egypt' *International Journal of Greek Love* Vol 1 No 1 (NY 1965).

Delacourt, Marie, *Hermaphodite* (London)

Dion Fortune, *Sane Occultism* (Aquarian Press 1987)

Dimock, D E, *The Hidden Moon*, (Rider).

Dimock, D. E.,. 'Goddess of Snakes in Medeival Bengali Literature' *Journal of the History of Religions*, (University of Chicago 1964).

Douglas, Nik and Slinger, Penny, *Sexual Secrets* (Arrow 1979).

Douglas, Mary, *Purity and Danger* (RKP 1978)

Eliade M., *Yoga, Immortality and Freedom* (Princeton 1969)

Ellman, Richard, *Yeats, The Man and the Masks* (Faber 1961)

Flescher Ronald, *Lecture Notes on Endocrinology* (Blackwell Scientific)

Foucault, Michel, *Herculine Barbine: being the recently discovered memoirs of a nineteenth century French hermaphrodite* (Harvester 1980) p. vii.

Goudrian, Teun and Gupta, Sanjukta *Hindu Tantrism* (Leiden, Brill)

Grant, Kenneth, *Aleister Crowley and the Hidden God* (Muller 1973)

Griffiths J. G., *The Contendings of Horus & Seth* (Liverpool UP 1960).

Hunt, A. S., 'An Incantation in the Ashmolean Museum' *Journal of Egyptian Archaeology* 15 1929 (p 155-157).

Sexual Magick

Iyengar, B K S., *Light on Yoga* (Allen & Unwin 1968)

Jung, C. G., 'Psychological Commentary on Kundalini Yoga' *Spring* 1975 & 1976.

Kant, I., *Dreams of a Spirit Seer*.

Kaulajnana Nirnaya, P C Bagchi (ed), translated into English by Mike Magee (Prachya Prakashan 1987).

King Francis, (Ed) *The Secret Rituals of the OTO* (Daniel 1973).

Kinsley, David, *Hindu Goddesses* (University of California Press 1986).

Knight, Gareth, *A Practical Guide to Qabalistic Symbolism* (Helios 1976)

Lane Fox, Robin, Pagans and Christians (Penguin 1986)

Lake Harris, T., *God's Breath in Man and in Humane Society: Law, Process and Result of Divine Natural Respiration* (Allen 1892).

Lake Harris, T.,*Wisdom of Angels - Poems* (New York 1857).

Lake Harris, T.,*The Marriage of Heaven & Earth* (Peace 1903)

Lake Harris, T., *The Triumph of Life* (Peace 1903).

Leslie, Charles, (ed) *Asian Medical Systems* (University of California Press 1976)

Liber Al, (Mandrake of Oxford 1993)

Lowen Alexander and Lowen, Leslie, *The Way to Vibrant Health* (Harper & Row 1977).

Lowndes Severly, Josephine, *Eve's Secrets* (London 1987)

Luhman, Tanya, *Persuasions of the Witch's Craft* (Blackwell 1989).

Martin, James, *Sexual Magick in Theory and Practice* (Abraxas 1993)

Mauss, Marcel, 'Body Techniques' in *Sociology and Psychology - Essays* (RKP:1979 London)

Monier-Williams, M., *Sanskrit-English Dictionary*, New Edition, (OUP 1979)

Morgan, Kris, *Medicine of the Gods* (Mandrake of Oxford 1994)

Morgan, Kris 'Catharsis' *Celtic Dawn* II Sept 1988.

Nuit Isis Reader, ed Katon Shual *et al* (Mandrake of Oxford 1994)

O'Flaherty, Wendy Doniger, Shiva: the Erotic-Ascetic, (OUP 1973) page 52.

O'Flaherty, Wendy D, *Hindu Myths* (Penguin 1975).

Overton-Fuller, J., *The Magical Dilemma of Victor Neuburg* (Mandrake of Oxford 1990)

Patanjali, *Yoga Sutras*, trans. R Prasada (Allahabad 1924)

Pingree, David 'History of Mathematical Astronomy in India' *Dictionary of Scientific Biography*, Vol 15, supp.1 (Scribners 1978)

Redgrove, Peter, *The Black Goddess and the Sixth Sense*, (Bloomsbury 1987)

Reich, Wilhelm, *The Function of the Orgasm*

Schäfer, Peter, *Gershom Scholem Reconsidered: the aim and purpose of early Jewish Mysticism*, (Oxford Centre for Postgraduate Hebrew Studies 1986.)

Scholem, Gershom, *Kabbalah* (New American Library 1974).

Shahidullah, *Dohakosha* No. 5

Shuttle, Penelope and Redgrove, Peter, *The Wise Wound - Menstruation and Everywoman* (1975)

Sircar S C., 'The Sakta Pithas', *Journal of the Royal Asiatic Society* (Bengal) Vol XIV 1948 pp. 1-108.

Starfire Magazine, edited by M Staley *et al.*

Swainson, W P., *Thomas Lake Harris and His Occult Teaching* (Rider 1922).

Taylor, Anne *L Oliphant* (OUP 1982)

Thelemic Magick XC (1994) - *Proceedings of the Ninth International Symposium of Thelemic Magick*, Snoo Wilson *et al* (Mandrake of Oxford 1995)

Velde H Te, *Seth - God of Confusion* (Leiden, Brill 1967).

Vogel, J Ph., *Indian Serpent Lore* (Probsthain 1926).

Walter, Michael L 'The Role of Alchemy and Medicine in Indo-Tibetan Tantrism' PhD Diss. 1980 (University of Indiana, Bloomington)

Wolff, Charlotte, *Magnus Hirschfeld - A Portrait of A Pioneer in Sexology* (Quartet 1986).

Wolff Charlotte, *Bisexuality* (Quartet)

Yeshe Tsogyal, *The Lotus Born - the life story of Padmasambhava* (Shambala 1993)

Zvelebil, K., *The Siddha Quest For Immortality* (Mandrake 1995).

Index

Agastya, 16
Ajna, 56
Akhanaten, 97
Alchemy, 45, 83
AMOOKOS, 52
    Tantra Magick, 63
Anahata, 56, 60
androgyny, 89
Argentinum Astrum, 11
Aristotle, 90
astrology, 102
auto-erotic magick, 33
Ayurveda, 18, 21, 72

Babalon, 29
Berridge, Edward 24
Besant, Annie 91
bisexuality, 31
Boddhicitta, 17
body magick, 50, 108
Book of Thoth, 76
Bornless One, 85
Buddhism, 11, 22, 101, 103, 101

chakras, 51, 60
    system of eleven 54
chastity, 88
Christianity, 87
circumambulation, 106, 109
confessional, 90

Confessions, 31
Crowley, Aleister 9, 26, 82, 91
De Arte Magica, 27
Eight Lectures on Yoga, 11
Liber Al, 29, 64, 76, 77
Liber O, 78
cunnilingus, 88

daath, 31
Daksa and the sacrifice, 100

Egypt, 85, 102
emotions, 60
endocrinology, 93

faecal products, 21
five 'Ms', 17
Farr Emery, Florence 25
Fortune, Dion 26, 40

Ganesha, 58, 68, 106
gender, 93
gentleness, 23
Goddess, 104
    dismembered, 104
Grant, Kenneth, 27, 70

Harris, Thomas Lake 14
Hermaphrodite, 93, 95
Hermetic Order of the Golden Dawn, 10, 23, 78

homosexuality, 13, 40, 77, 82, 87, 89
human sacrifice, 103

kalas, 27, 70
Kali, 105
Kalyanamalla's *Anangaranga*, 70
Kama Sutra, 10, 70
Kamarupa, 58, 63, 101
    Temple Meditation, 64
karezza, 14
Kenneth Grant, 27, 62
    Aleister Crowley and the Hidden God, 77
Knight, Gareth 42
Kundalini, 51, 56, 59, 62, 63

Leadbeater, C W 52
Lesbians, 43
Light On Yoga, 61
lingams, 104
Lopamudra, 16

Mathers, MacGregor 24
Magia Sexualis, 10
Manipura, 55, 60
marriage, 87, 90
martial arts, 11
Matsyendranath, 103
Melusina, 59
menstruation, 32
muladhara, 54, 58

Nagas, 59
Nath Clan, 52
Neuberg, Victor 11, 82
Nuit, 58, 80
nyasa, 69, 107

ojas, 21
orgasm, 91
OTO, 28
Oxyrhynchus fish, 102

Parched Grain, 20
Paris Working, 82
passivity, 88
pilgrimage, 98, 106
pilgrimage, internal, 107
Pitha, 99, 100
porn, 19
Pythagoreans, 88

Rasa, 45
Rasaratnakâra, 83
Reich, Wilhelm
    The Function of the Orgasm, 73
Rig Veda, 17
ritual, 62
ritual intercourse, 16
rivers, 108
    shrines, 107

sacred, 57
sadhaka, 102
Sahajayana, 101

Sahajiyas, 48
sahasrara, 56
sandhyâbhâshâ, 17
Sankhya, 52
Sati, 100
seat of goddess see pitha, 100
semen, 90
    loss, 22
    female, 90
sensual enjoyment, 87
Serpent Power, The 51
Seth, 76, 80, 82, 84, 102, 104
    Seth and Horus, 80
    Seth spell, 84
sexual mores, 87
Shiva, 100
Shri Yantra, 10
solar plexus, 53
spirit of place, 98
spleen, 53
Sprinkle, Annie 19
Steinach therapy, 25
Stele of Revealing, 79

Stoicism, 87
svadhisthana, 55, 60

tantra, 12, 101, 107
Taoism, 11
Tetratis, 64
Theatre of Memory, 64
Thelema, 11, 30
Theosophical Society, 10, 53
Typhon, 84

uddiyana, 21, 102
urine, 18

Vajroli Mudra, 21
Vaughan, Thomas 45
vishuddha, 56, 60

Wise Wound, The 32

Yeats, W B 25
Yoga, 11, 24, 61
    Yogasutras, 89